HOW TO SLEEP

HOW TO
SLEEP

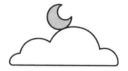

The New Science-Based Solutions
for Sleeping Through the Night

RAFAEL PELAYO, MD

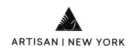

ARTISAN | NEW YORK

Dedicated to the legacy of my friend William Dement,
who made the world a better place

Library of Congress Cataloging-in-Publication Data

Name: Pelayo, Rafael, author.
Title: How to sleep : the new science-based solutions for sleeping through the night /
　　Rafael Pelayo, MD
Description: New York : Artisan Books, a division of Workman Publishing Co., Inc., [2020] |
　　Includes index.
Identifiers: LCCN 2020020140 | ISBN 9781579659578 (hardcover)
Subjects: LCSH: Sleep—Popular works. | Sleep disorders—Treatment—Popular works.
Classification: LCC RA786 .P44 2020 | DDC 616.8/498—dc23
LC record available at https://lccn.loc.gov/2020020140

Design by Nina Simoneaux

Artisan books are available at special discounts when purchased in bulk for premiums and sales promotions as well as for fund-raising or educational use. Special editions or book excerpts also can be created to specification. For details, contact the Special Sales Director at the address below, or send an e-mail to specialmarkets@workman.com.

For speaking engagements, contact speakersbureau@workman.com.

Published by Artisan
A division of Workman Publishing Co., Inc.
225 Varick Street
New York, NY 10014-4381
artisanbooks.com

Artisan is a registered trademark of Workman Publishing Co., Inc.

Published simultaneously in Canada by Thomas Allen & Son, Limited

Printed in China

First printing, November 2020

10 9 8 7 6 5 4 3 2 1

CONTENTS

INTRODUCTION

EVERYBODY SLEEPS. In fact, you've been sleeping longer than you've been eating food or breathing air. (We may even dream in the weeks before we are born.) Sleep science pioneer Dr. Allan Rechtschaffen once said, "If sleep has no function, it is the biggest mistake made by evolution." It's no mistake: Though the functions of sleep have long been considered a mystery, scientific data increasingly show that sleep is how humans' bodies and brains are restored and recharged. Our metabolisms require it. Little wonder that we wake up feeling cranky and unfocused when we don't sleep well. Nothing consistently makes you feel better than a good night of sleep.

But on any given night, about half of us think we don't sleep well. Routinely waking up feeling irritable and tired is the first sign that you may have a sleep problem. Sleep difficulties affect millions of people—and the problem is getting worse. The Centers for Disease Control and Prevention has described sleep disorders as an epidemic in our society.

You can sleep better. And after reading this book, you *will* sleep better. As a sleep-medicine physician, I can say that with confidence. In my more than twenty-five years of practice, I've seen again and again that sleep patients are capable of major improvement—so long as they're given the right "rules" to follow.

The Old Rules Don't Work

News stories about this "sleep epidemic" often conclude with a similar litany of advice referred to collectively since the 1970s as "sleep hygiene" rules. The term sleep hygiene, widely used by both health professionals and the general public, refers to isolated recommendations of things to avoid, such as "Don't read in bed," "Don't drink coffee close to bedtime," "Don't watch TV in bed," and "Don't drink alcohol before bedtime." The concept, popularized by the late great Dr. Peter Hauri, was well-intentioned and has helped generate awareness of the importance of sleep. But despite the popularity of these old rules, improving one's sleep hygiene alone is rarely effective in helping people with serious sleep problems.

In my practice, I've found that sleep hygiene rules are a well-meaning but simplistic shortcut approach to difficulties in sleeping. Expecting sleep hygiene alone to help a person with chronic sleep difficulties is like telling somebody with an anxiety disorder to stop worrying. Almost every new patient I see tells me they already practice sleep hygiene. Many of these patients are able to recite the usual sleep hygiene rules backward and forward, but they *still* have trouble sleeping. Despite knowing these rules for decades, millions of people continue to battle sleep difficulties.

The data collected so far back me up: According to the American Academy of Sleep Medicine, research clearly shows that the efficacy of sleep hygiene rules alone is weak and inconclusive at best. This is because applying those rules ignores the core issues that cause sleep disorders. If anything, it can backfire, because when people try to use sleep hygiene rules and still sleep poorly, they blame themselves or become resigned to poor sleep because they've "tried everything." It's a kitchen-sink approach that fails to address each person's specific issues.

The New Sleep Rules

Based on my years of clinical experience with patients, scientific research, and community outreach work, I know that people can develop better, smarter, long-lasting sleep patterns. What follows are a new set of rules designed to reflect the growth of knowledge in sleep science and offer a clear path to effectively improving your health. It all begins with making quality sleep a priority, which you've already begun to do, just by opening up this book!

In chapter one we'll take a step back and I'll explain how sleep works as part of our biology, why we sleep, and how sleep is essential for our waking life. I have found that putting people's personal sleep challenges in context quickly changes their perspective. In chapter two we'll take a deep dive into the most common physical impediments to good-quality sleep (beginning with snoring). In chapter three I'll discuss the tips and tools to help rid yourself of insomnia once and for all, and in chapter four I'll not only address how everyday lifestyle choices (such as what we eat and drink and how we exercise) affect sleep, but also take a clear-eyed look at sleep remedies that work—and those that don't. A brief survey of troubling but less common sleep disorders like sleepwalking and narcolepsy follows in chapter five, and because it is never too soon or too late to learn how to improve your sleep, in chapter six I'll offer strategies that apply to infants, seniors, and everyone in between. Chapter seven tackles the wondrous realm of dreams and the exciting science behind the miracle of the sleeping mind.

If, after reading the preceding chapters, you still have trouble sleeping or feel you need some extra help to resolve your sleep difficulties, then you may need to see a sleep-medicine physician. In chapter eight I'll guide you through a virtual visit to a sleep doctor to show you how a combination of state-of-the-art technology and old-fashioned medical sleuthing can help determine what exactly is disrupting your sleep.

The information in this book will help you sleep better, wake up refreshed, and have a healthier life. It's time to put the sleep-disorder epidemic to bed.

ONE

HOW SLEEP WORKS

BEFORE YOU CAN sleep better (and you *will* sleep better), you need to understand the biology of normal sleep. Early scientists believed that sleep was little more than an inactive state. It wasn't until brain-wave activity could be reliably monitored that we discovered that our journey through the night is fascinating and complex—and far from inactive. There is a lot going on while we're sleeping, and scientific studies of the sleeping brain are revealing not only how the human organism functions during sleep but also how our sleep affects us while we're awake. The mystery of sleep is no longer so mysterious.

Circadian Rhythms

Inside our heads is what's known as the circadian or biological clock. This miniature timekeeper consists of a tiny cluster of neurons that shares one purpose: to synchronize the body's biological rhythms with the earth's cycles of dawn and dusk.

This clock is located in the perfect place: at the base of the brain, right behind our eyes and above the junction of our optic nerves, which transmit information to the circadian clock about the light that is coming into our eyes. (The fact that this small region has the best blood supply in the entire brain underscores its vital importance. A person who suffers a major stroke is much more likely to lose their ability to speak or move their hand than suffer damage to their circadian clock!)

The circadian clock's internal rhythm runs slightly longer than twenty-four hours, to predict the incremental changes in the earth's rotational tilt that affect the length of our days and nights across the seasons, so it tends to overshoot. But it resets at the first burst of light to hit our eyes when we wake in the morning. Once the brain knows what time the light hits our eyes, it can predict that dawn will occur around the same time the next day. This is essential to our survival: In our ancient past, if we left the safety of the village or caves we lived in, we had to ensure we'd be back to our homes before dusk, when nocturnal predators became active. But if we left too late or returned too early, we wasted potential daylight to hunt and gather.

Our circadian clock sends us signals to begin the process of falling asleep as nighttime comes, and it emits chemicals to naturally wake us up as dawn approaches. Our goal should be to work *with* this clock instead of fight against it.

Because our sleep patterns are influenced by light, it's not surprising that seasonality has an effect on our sleep needs. These changes are usually too subtle to be noticeable, but if you live nearer to the poles, like in Alaska, where the amount of light varies drastically between seasons, you may sleep more in winter and less in summer. With the prevalence of artificial light, many of us are trapped into thinking it's always a short summer night and end up sleeping as little as possible! (This is why it's important to control your light situation for optimal sleep wherever you are—see page 76 for more.)

You Are Most Awake Before You Go to Sleep

If sleep worked like the fuel in a car, then we would be most alert when we first wake up and become less and less alert throughout the day—just like cars' tanks are at their maximum capacity right after we fill them with fuel and get depleted the longer we drive. But sleep and alertness work in a more complex way.

Most of us wake up somewhat sleepy, even if we've had a normal, restful night's sleep. We become more alert as the morning goes on. We may begin to feel drowsy again in the afternoon (and no, the culprit is not your lunch—consider that neither breakfast nor dinner makes us very sleepy). If we can shake off our afternoon slump, in the evening we will find ourselves feeling more alert than we were earlier in the day even though our "tank" is nearly empty.

The reason for this is that while the pressure to sleep builds the longer we stay awake, our circadian clock sends an alerting signal to the brain to counter this pressure. This signal is most powerful about two hours before we normally go to sleep. This accounts for the "second wind" many people claim to experience at night. It also explains why it is easier to stay up late than it is to go to sleep earlier than usual.

This circadian modulation of sleepiness and alertness helped ensure our survival: We are most alert close to bedtime because this is when our former predators, like lions and tigers, are on the hunt. We balance this peak of alertness with a lull when the day is at its hottest and predators are having a lull of their own. The clock in our heads is a truly amazing legacy of our evolution.

Sleep Is an Active Process

My patients often say they have trouble sleeping because they "can't turn off their brains." But as long as we are alive and healthy, our brains are not meant to be turned off!

For centuries, sleep was considered a passive, almost deathlike state. But with the advent of modern sleep science, we now know that sleep is an active process. The brain is not turned off but instead goes through predictable cycles of various sleep patterns known as sleep stages. The repetitive combination of sleep stages is referred to as a person's sleep architecture.

The modern era of sleep science was born in the 1950s when scientists began combining measurements of brain waves with other electrical signals from the body. To help make sense of the measurements, scientists divided sleep into two distinct modes: rapid eye movement (REM) sleep and non–rapid eye movement (NREM) sleep. Since 75 to 80 percent of our sleep time is in

NREM, scientists further divide it into three stages that correspond to light, intermediate, and deep sleep (N1, N2, and N3, respectively).

Many significant things occur during NREM, including the physical growth of our bodies and memory consolidation. NREM sleep is even thought to have a key function in the restoration of our brains by resetting our brain synapses. In NREM we have our deepest sleep.

In the N1 period of NREM sleep, we transition from the awake state into sleep. We become much less aware of the outside world as we turn inward. Our eyes close and start to slowly roll back in our heads. In this drowsy state, we may think we are still awake, but anyone watching us can see we are checking out.

In N2, which takes up about half of our total sleep time, we have bursts of unique brain-wave patterns called sleep spindles and K-complexes. Sleep spindles are thought to play a role in the brain forming declarative, or explicit, memories—memories of facts and occurrences that can be consciously recalled, such as specific events in our lives or new information we learned that day.

N3 (commonly referred to as slow-wave sleep) is our deepest sleep. Dominating the first third of the night, N3 takes up 10 percent or less of total adult sleep time (children and teenagers will have as much as 20 percent and sometimes even more N3 sleep). In N3, our breathing and heart rate reach their lowest point. This is the period when it is the most difficult to wake us up. N3 is when our brains secrete the most growth hormone (and likely the time when children's bones actually grow longer—inadequate sleep is associated with growth problems in children). It, too, is thought to play a role in consolidating our memories and may be a future target for therapies for conditions such as dementia. In

N3, odd phenomena such as sleepwalking can occur (see page 90 for more).

REM is the sleep stage most closely associated with dreaming and dominates the last third of the night. Looking solely at brain waves, it is difficult to distinguish REM sleep from being awake, with our eyes open. This implies that the mental activity of looking around while awake and dreaming are similar. (In contrast, when we are awake with our eyes closed, our brain waves look completely different.) Although most of our other muscles stop moving, our eye movements dramatically change as we transition from NREM into REM, with wild, seemingly chaotic movements (hence the name). Our heart rates also fluctuate greatly. If you lead a sedentary lifestyle, REM may be when you reach your peak heart rate on a given day. REM episodes tend to become longer in later sleep cycles, and at the end of the REM bouts, we usually change our sleeping positions and briefly wake up (more on this on page 18).

Each complete sleep cycle—which can include all of the NREM and REM stages—lasts about ninety minutes, although individual cycles vary throughout the night. As shown in the illustration opposite, we sleep most deeply in the early cycles, and REM is longer and more intense in the later cycles. The first sleep cycle is dominated by our deep, slow-wave sleep and contains very little REM sleep. As the night goes on, this mixture changes, so that by the early-morning hours we have very little of that deep sleep, and REM sleep prevails. (This is why we have our longest and most intense dreams just before we wake up to start our day.)

This overall pattern of sleep stages and cycles—your sleep architecture—reflects the quality of your sleep. Many potential clues into people's sleep problems can be found by analyzing their sleep architecture (for example, see You Should Never Wake Up Tired, page 25).

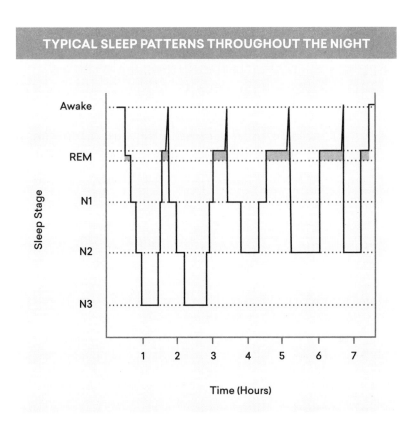

All Sleep Stages Are Created Equal

You might assume that because slow-wave (N3) sleep helps our bodies and minds recover and reenergize, it is the most important, most refreshing sleep of the night. It is important, and it is refreshing, but as discussed on page 15, slow-wave sleep makes up only about 10 percent of total sleep time in healthy adults. Does that mean that 90 percent of sleep isn't as necessary? Clearly this is not the case. If slow-wave sleep was the only sleep you got at night, you would feel the full effects of sleep deprivation.

I'm often asked what the most important sleep stage is. Behind this question, I suspect, is a hope that perhaps there is a stage of sleep we can do without. If we could replace our light sleep with deeper sleep, maybe we'd feel more refreshed when we wake up. It remains to be seen if this is possible to do safely or in any sustained way.

In fact, our brains have some self-correction with regard to our sleep stages. If, for example, we wake up too early and cut off some of our REM time, when we do get a chance to sleep again, we will have more REM sleep than usual. This is called REM pressure and explains why when we are very sleep deprived we may start to dream with our eyes open.

No One Sleeps through the Night

Each of us wakes up about every ninety minutes in our sleep cycle. We toss, stir, change position, sometimes even open our eyes and scan the room. It's a phenomenon so brief (lasting less than a minute) that in most instances we don't remember doing it. Not only do we wake up at ninety-minute intervals, but about ten times an hour we have short arousals lasting approximately three seconds each. In all of these instances, your brain is simply doing what it is supposed to do. If we slept straight through for seven or eight hours in a row, the lions and tigers would have picked us off into extinction long ago! Waking up during the night is normal; having trouble going back to sleep is not. No matter how sleepless you feel, make this your mantra: *Sleep will come.* It's a natural function of human biology.

Sleep Fragmentation: Stuck in First Gear

More than any specific sleep stage, what matters for refreshing sleep is the healthy continuity of the sleep cycles. When these cycles are disrupted, we use the term sleep fragmentation. Think of the natural mixture of sleep stages as your car's transmission. The normal progression of shifting gears (moving from one sleep stage to the next) allows you to efficiently obtain a smooth ride (a good night's sleep). But if your transmission is slipping (continuously starting and stopping your sleep), or you're stuck in first gear (N1 sleep), you will have an inefficient and choppy ride—you're not getting the good sleep you need.

Your sleep fragmentation may be out of your control; it could be the fault of a snoring sleep partner or a crying infant, or a painful condition that wakes you in the night. There might not be much you can do to prevent these sorts of interruptions (short of getting your partner to a sleep doctor—see page 136!). But there are some behaviors you *can* curtail, such as drinking alcohol or caffeine close to bedtime or taking long naps during the day, to prevent sleep fragmentation.

You Might Not Need Eight Hours of Sleep

An average of seven to eight hours of sleep allows most people to wake up feeling their best, but the optimal number of hours one should sleep depends on the individual and the assumptions that your sleep is normal in quality and its timing is predictable. Ultimately, there's no magic number of hours you need to sleep each night. Put simply, you need as many hours of sleep as it takes for you to wake up feeling refreshed and remain alert throughout the day. "Short sleepers" seem to have a genetic predisposition to sleep fewer hours than average, while "long sleepers" tend to need more sleep. But if your need for sleep noticeably changes, consult a doctor.

Can I Get By with Less Sleep?

You can't. Next question.

Seriously, Can I Get By with Less Sleep?

A fortune is waiting for anyone who can come up with a way to give us the restorative effects of eight hours of sleep in only four hours. You may be able to "get by" with less sleep than your body requires, but you are doing only that, getting by. The ability to put off sleep is built into our brains, and we can do it up to a point. We can also skip meals—our physiology has evolved to allow us to temporarily go without the basic necessities. But we do not function at our best in these situations. For optimum mental and physical health, don't treat sleep like an inconvenience; make it a priority in your life.

What Happens When We Don't Sleep?

Sleep consumes one-third of our lives, and poor sleep can severely impair the other two-thirds. It's essential for our health and wellness. Just consider what happens when someone *doesn't* sleep: After just twenty-four hours without sleep, a person's reaction time is similar to that of a drunk driver. When we are fighting to stay awake, we may have brief bouts of sleep called microsleeps, where we might not even realize we have fallen asleep—a potentially dangerous situation if we're driving or operating machinery. Going even longer without any sleep, known as complete sleep deprivation, makes a person increasingly irritable, emotional, and inattentive. Reaction time is further diminished. After not sleeping for three days or more, a person may start to hallucinate and eventually become delirious.

Suffering from poor-quality sleep for an extended period of time can have the same general effects as complete sleep deprivation, putting yourself and others at risk during unconscious microsleeps. It's perhaps even more dangerous, because people with chronic sleep deprivation may be unaware of the effects that lack of sleep is having on them. There are many serious physical, psychological, and emotional tolls caused by extended periods of poor sleep. Long-standing sleep deprivation is a stressor on the body, and it is not only associated with a greater risk of obesity, diabetes, hypertension, and cardiovascular disease, but also may increase the risk of cancer and serious neurological conditions such as Alzheimer's. Significant cognitive deficits can occur, including decreased thinking speed and verbal memory, and even a greater likelihood of forming false memories! Your mood may suffer, you may overreact to stressful situations, and you are more likely to engage in risky and impulsive behavior. If you suffer from mental illness, lack of sleep can exacerbate these conditions. Simply put, we have to sleep well to be healthy.

Sleep and Immunity

If you deprive yourself of sleep, your body's immune system cannot function at its best. Lack of sleep is a stressor to the body, and the body's reaction to this stress is similar to its response to low-grade inflammation.

Common wisdom has it that when you feel sick, you should take to your bed. In fact, the release of special immune-system proteins called cytokines—part of the body's reaction to infection—makes you sleepy, so bed rest is often just what the doctor ordered. If you don't get the necessary sleep when you're fighting off an illness, you are adding to the demands of your body to mount an anti-inflammatory reaction. So if you get sick, don't try to work your way through it.

You should also be prioritizing sleep *before* you get sick, as sleep deprivation makes us more prone to getting infections in the first place. Lack of sleep interferes with the immune system's T-cells, which help us fight infections caused by viruses. This is likely one of the reasons we get colds so easily when we travel and our sleep patterns are out of whack. Even healthy young people, if sleep deprived, will become ill more frequently (which may be one of the reasons so many partying spring breakers get sick and why younger people can become sicker than expected if they contract an illness such as COVID-19).

As discussed on page 20, we don't all require the same amount of sleep each night, but one study showed that people who reported habitually sleeping only five hours per night had an increased risk for developing pneumonia in the next two years, and a higher incidence of respiratory infection in the previous month when compared with people who usually slept seven to eight hours per night. (Interestingly, participants reporting five hours of sleep a night who felt their sleep duration was adequate did not have an increased pneumonia risk—meaning these findings can be better generalized for people who are not getting as much sleep as their bodies need.)

The good news is that regularly getting a good night's sleep can actually *boost* our immune systems, with measurably reduced risk of infections and improved infection outcomes. Even our bodies' response to vaccinations is affected by our sleep! Sleep really is the ultimate form of self-care.

Can I Catch Up on Sleep?

When we don't get enough sleep, that missing sleep does not just go away. It accumulates, just like any other debt. For example, if your daily sleep requirement is seven hours, sleeping five hours a night for one five-day workweek will create a sleep debt of ten hours. The larger the sleep debt, the stronger the tendency to fall asleep during the day and to feel fatigued, among other potential ills.

The only known way to pay off sleep debt? Sleep. Returning to our example: Let's say you sleep in on Saturday after your week of late nights. This might chip away at your ten-hour sleep debt, but it won't be effective in *eliminating* that debt. The only way to truly "pay off" your sleep debt is to change the habits that led you to accumulate it in the first place.

Can I Get Too Much Sleep?

There's no evidence that "too much sleep" is a legitimate phenomenon. Still, anyone who sleeps for an unusually long period of time—whether a student sleeping off an all-nighter or a shift worker coming off a twenty-four-hour workday—can wake up feeling groggy, achy, and listless, the opposite of refreshed and alert.

The explanation for this is threefold: First, the ability to sleep twelve hours or more indicates a very large sleep debt, which simply can't be eliminated in one extended sleep period—it may take a week or so to get back to normal. Second, when you sleep until midday or into the afternoon, you're waking up close to the classic midday drowsy slump, and the timing of your body's hormones will be out of sync with their usual rhythm. Third, a long period of immobility can result in muscle aches or stiffness.

Alas, while you can accumulate sleep debt, you cannot store up sleep. A normal, predictable sleep pattern should be the goal each and every night.

You Should Never Wake Up Tired

You don't leave a satisfying meal feeling hungry, so why should you wake up from a full night's sleep feeling tired and groggy? A good sleep means waking up feeling refreshed. If you wake up tired no matter how much you sleep, then you should talk to your doctor about options to accurately measure the *quality* of your sleep.

It is likely that you are getting too much N1 sleep. This stage is how we naturally enter sleep and is the lightest sleep you can have. Think of it as the first gear in your car's transmission. You could drive your car across the entire country in first gear, but it would be inefficient and prevent your car from performing optimally. In the same way, sleeping through the night in N1 will leave you feeling tired. People with chronic pain, for example, often have excess N1 sleep, enduring nights of choppy or continually interrupted sleep (see Sleep Fragmentation: Stuck in First Gear, page 19).

An overnight sleep study—spending a night in a sleep lab being monitored by medical staff—is often the best way to get to the bottom of your poor-quality sleep. For more on this, see page 144.

Will I Go Crazy If I Don't Sleep?

You won't go crazy if you go too long without sleep, but you can become temporarily delirious (among other serious side effects— see page 21). Sleep deprivation can be dangerous, but it doesn't cause permanent insanity. This has actually been tested. For many years one of the pioneers of REM sleep, Dr. William Dement, tried to use sleep deprivation as a scientific model to study schizophrenia. It didn't pan out. Even though heavily sleep-deprived persons can have delirious thoughts and may even hallucinate, once you leave them alone and let them sleep, they'll return to their usual (sane) self.

Night Owls versus Morning Larks

Our circadian clock is regulated by genes we inherit from our parents. Variations among these genes predict who identifies as a morning lark and who is more of a night owl. These variations are not always obvious in young children, who have a hard time staying awake much past their usual (and usually well-enforced) bedtime. It's during adolescence when the night owls tend to emerge.

But genes are only part of the story. Rats are nocturnal, having a sleeping pattern that allows them to avoid daytime predators. If you captured a wild rat and only fed it during the day, initially the rat would go hungry. But gradually it would learn that it's safe to eat during the day, and this genetically nocturnal animal would become more active by day (diurnal). What does this mean for us? That our tendencies are not our destiny! A night owl can adjust to an early-morning exercise routine, and a morning lark can adjust to working the night shift.

The lines blur further the older we get, when it becomes harder to stay up late, whether we're affirmed night owls or morning larks. This may be related to hormonal changes in the way our bodies handle melatonin. Another possible contributor: changes in our vision. As we age, less light reaches our retinas, weakening the effects of light on our circadian rhythms; new studies show that people who undergo cataract surgery report sleeping better with their newly implanted lenses.

Both biological and learned factors play a role in our sleep preferences, and understanding the principles guiding our sleep can help us adapt to our changing environments.

The Skinny on "Second Sleep"

Also known as polyphasic sleep, second sleep is the habit of breaking up your nighttime sleep into two parts, with a period of activity in between. Though it's become trendy in the digital information age, it's not a new phenomenon. Historical evidence shows that early humans, especially those living in agrarian societies, took advantage of the cooler nighttime hours to get work done between a first and second sleep. As the modern age dawned and nine-to-five work schedules became the norm, sleeping in a single block of time seemed more efficient, and humans adjusted to this sleep pattern.

These days, with the gig economy making work schedules more flexible, we are seeing a resurgence of interest in second sleep. From a biological standpoint, humans are certainly capable of shifting to a second-sleep schedule: We routinely awaken briefly during the night at the end of each sleep cycle anyway (see page 18). But being out of sync with the schedules of family, friends, and coworkers or clients may prove impractical. My personal choice for a polyphasic sleep period? A luxurious, old-fashioned nap.

Sleep Is Delicious

Few things in life are more satisfying than waking up refreshed after a full night of sleep. It really is . . . delicious! Sleep is an appetitive behavior, meaning we have a natural desire to satisfy our need for sleep. And the area of the brain that regulates hunger and eating, the hypothalamus, is also very much involved in the basic regulation of our sleep. In experiments, when an animal is sleep deprived, it will eat more. When humans don't get enough sleep, they tend not only to seek out food but also to make more impulsive food choices. You may find that a brief nap is more satisfying than any big lunch!

You Will Always Sleep

Human sleep is homeostatic, meaning that it is a system that seeks balance. The more time you spend awake, the more you need to sleep. As long as you are alive, you cannot indefinitely stop yourself from sleeping—that would be like voluntarily trying to hold your breath. Eventually your biology will force you to breathe again. And so it goes with sleep. It's a natural process, one people with insomnia should take to heart: As a homeostatic function of the brain, sleep *will* eventually return.

TWO

SNORING? START HERE

BEFORE YOU CAN address any behavioral or environmental factors that may be affecting your sleep, you need to rule out physical ones. If you snore, it's critical to determine if sleep-disordered breathing and obstructive sleep apnea (the interruption of breathing during sleep) are at the root of your sleep problem. Obstructive sleep apnea is incredibly common; it's the disorder we see most in sleep-medicine clinics. This chapter is a brief overview of sleep apnea and other common physical conditions that might be impacting your sleep, which should be addressed with the help of a sleep clinician.

It's Never Normal to Snore

We all know the sounds of snoring, from the repetitive, sawlike "cutting z's" to the occasional sudden snort. Snoring during sleep is common, but it is also a red flag that something is wrong. People don't snore when they're awake, after all. Why, from an evolutionary standpoint, would we tip off our presence to predators when our guard is down? Snoring would be a dinner bell!

It's common to snore in transient situations—such as when recovering from a cold, for example—but otherwise *sleeping should be silent*. The sounds of snoring indicate that some kind of abnormal airflow obstruction or turbulence is causing you to have difficulty breathing, forcing you to mouth breathe in your sleep. It's a simple concept: If you don't get enough air in through your nose, your mouth will drop open. This often happens when we exercise. It should not happen when you sleep.

Snoring can be measured or tracked in different ways, but the easiest may be simply by asking a bed partner, who sees and hears (practically) all. But what if you sleep alone? How do you know if you snore? If you find yourself waking frequently in the night with a dry mouth or needing to drink water, it may indicate that you are mouth breathing in your sleep. If you occasionally share sleeping space with a friend or family member (while traveling, for example), give that person permission to let you know if you snore. Or simply record yourself as you sleep during the night.

If you do snore, don't ignore it. Tell your health-care provider. If your health-care provider tells you not to worry about it because they snore, too, get a new doctor! And if you hear someone snoring, let them know. You might be saving their life.

The first step in correcting snoring is determining if you suffer from simple snoring (see Other Snoring Solutions, page 36) or the more serious obstructive sleep apnea.

Obstructive Sleep Apnea

The word apnea means "absence of breathing," and a sleep apnea episode occurs when someone stops breathing during sleep. Plainly speaking, during a sleep apnea episode, sleeping is momentarily more important than breathing to your brain.

It is a potentially serious disorder, and yet it's incredibly common: Some thirty million Americans suffer from obstructive sleep apnea. The cardinal symptoms are fatigue and snoring, but the disorder can also induce heart attacks and strokes. Apnea's disruptions to sleep alone can cause behavioral changes and memory or learning problems. The good news is, obstructive sleep apnea may well be one of the most treatable health-care problems in the country. One of the most common (and successful) remedies for sleep apnea is the nightly use of a CPAP machine (see page 33); other options include an oral mouthpiece, corrective surgery, or—if your obstructive sleep apnea is relatively mild—behavioral fixes such as losing weight, not sleeping on your back, or avoiding alcohol close to bedtime (see page 60).

To test for sleep apnea, you will need to have a sleep study. Increasingly, patients bring in their own recordings of their snoring, but insurance companies typically will not pay for the treatment of sleep apnea unless the condition is confirmed with a sleep test. There are various ways to measure for sleep apnea, and emerging technology is further adding to our diagnostic options. It's even allowing sleep studies to be done in a person's home. (For more on sleep studies, see page 144.)

The sleep study is administered during the time a person typically sleeps, for most people overnight. This all-night sleep recording is called a polysomnogram (PSG). A PSG measures a person's brain waves, eye movements, body movements, muscle tone, breathing patterns, oxygen levels, and heart rhythm. For the diagnosis of obstructive sleep apnea, the recording will add up how often the patient either stopped breathing entirely (apneas) or had episodes of shallow breathing that resulted in drops in oxygen levels and disrupted sleep (hypopneas). The total number of apneas and hypopneas during the night divided by the total hours of sleep is calculated as the apnea-hypopnea index (AHI). If the AHI is greater than five events per hour, the diagnosis of sleep apnea is confirmed. An AHI of greater than thirty indicates severe sleep apnea.

Overlooked, sleep apnea may complicate the treatment of other health problems. Doctors often see patients with complex medical situations and myriad complaints that are hard to sort into a single, clear diagnosis. Sleep apnea acts like a fog, getting in the way of clearly seeing what else is going on with the patient. If you have concerns about snoring or feel chronically fatigued or sleepy in the daytime, consult your doctor about getting tested for sleep apnea. Address your sleep apnea, and you may find that treatments that previously failed for other ailments now work! When obstructive sleep apnea is remedied, you really get a fresh start.

CPAP Will Turbo-Charge Your Sleep

When we fall asleep, the muscles in our throat relax and our airway can become too narrow, making it harder to inflate our lungs. The work of breathing increases, and we have to create more negative pressure to inhale. It's like trying to drink a milkshake through a very thin straw. A cascade of events can ensue, culminating in obstructive sleep apnea and all of its potential dire consequences.

A CPAP (continuous positive airway pressure) machine is a bedside device successfully used by millions of people to treat obstructive sleep apnea. A CPAP machine features a hose with a mask that forces positive pressure through your nose. This positive pressure counteracts the negative pressure that is causing your airway to implode when you have obstructive sleep apnea. The invention of the CPAP machine was inspired by reversing the flow of a vacuum cleaner, and the original CPAP machines were just as loud as those household appliances. Modern CPAP devices, however, are nearly silent. They are certainly quieter than snoring!

Using a CPAP machine can be a game changer for your health and well-being. Most patients are astounded at how much better they feel when they use CPAP devices; they feel rejuvenated, their memory may improve, and their libido often increases. Yet many people struggle with wearing the device, become frustrated, and give up, often blaming themselves. Does wearing a mask over your face or nose while sleeping take some getting used to? Undoubtedly. But if I sold you a pair of shoes and they gave you blisters, would you blame the shoes or your feet? If you have sleep apnea and CPAP makes you feel worse, the problem is not likely to be you, but rather the equipment. First, make sure the mask is the right size for you by trying out a number of models. Some are nasal masks; full-face masks cover your nose and mouth. If you continue to snore while wearing a CPAP machine, it has not been set up correctly. Your snoring should be completely gone when the device is working properly.

If you have tried CPAP in the past and had trouble with it, talk to a board-certified sleep physician about trying it again. These devices have never been smaller, quieter, or more effective than they are now. The latest "smart CPAPs" are computerized devices that correct obstructed breathing episodes on a breath-by-breath basis. When you wake up, a smart CPAP tells you how well you slept and how effective the treatment was, and it can even transmit this information wirelessly to your physician, who can change device settings remotely.

But I Don't Want a CPAP Machine!

If you have obstructive sleep apnea, you owe it to yourself to give the CPAP treatment option a proper try. A CPAP machine is effective and probably the best bang for your buck—but it's not for everyone. Fortunately, there are several alternative options.

An oral appliance can treat obstructive sleep apnea by moving the tongue to create more space to breathe. There are dozens of varieties of oral appliances on the market; look for those custom-made by dentists trained in the treatment of obstructive sleep apnea. Oral appliance treatments have the advantage of being more discreet than a CPAP machine. Looking much like boxers' mouthpieces, they don't require electricity and are easy to travel with. But a custom-made oral appliance can be considerably more expensive than a CPAP machine, and oral appliances address obstructive sleep apnea only at the level of the tongue, meaning they may not be fully effective when someone has additional levels of obstruction (such as in the soft palate or nose area). Since many oral appliances move the jaw, they can also sometimes cause pain in the temporomandibular joint (TMJ) area or throw off the alignment of a person's teeth. If you're interested in using an oral appliance, you'll need a repeat sleep study to ensure that the device is truly effective, as well as regular visits to the dentist to make sure the device is working correctly and your teeth are not becoming misaligned. All of this adds to the cost of treatment, but many people who wish to avoid a CPAP machine swear by oral appliances.

Surgery was the primary treatment for obstructive sleep apnea until the mid-1980s when CPAP became available, and a number of surgical approaches are very effective. In children, removal of the tonsils and adenoids usually resolves the issue. For adults, very sophisticated and effective surgeries exist that rearrange the lower facial bones to correct the actual anatomical problem causing the obstruction. There are also implantable pacemaker-like devices that can synchronize to your breathing while awake to move the tongue out of the way and relieve the obstruction during sleep. But be aware that there are other painful and relatively ineffective surgical approaches that merely reduce snoring—I compare these to turning off a fire alarm instead of putting out the fire.

For many people with obstructive sleep apnea, weight loss is an effective solution. The good news is that losing a relatively small amount of weight can have a big impact on your breathing while you sleep. Many people, especially men, put on weight around the neck, narrowing the throat area and obstructing breathing. Losing roughly 10 to 15 percent of your body weight can drastically open up the space in the throat area and help you breathe better at night. The bad news is that for these same reasons, relatively small increases in weight can lead to disproportionate worsening of the obstruction. (It's important to note, though, that not only overweight people suffer from sleep apnea!)

If your obstructive sleep apnea is relatively mild, you may be able to resolve it with behavioral fixes like avoiding alcohol close to bedtime or not sleeping on your back. That said, positional therapy devices—gadgets marketed to obstructive sleep apnea sufferers to help prevent them from sleeping on their backs—may initially reduce snoring, but because obstructive sleep apnea tends to gradually worsen over time as people age or gain weight, positional devices are often ineffective long term.

Many obstructive sleep apnea treatments can be combined. For example, a person may use a CPAP machine at home but turn to an oral appliance when they are traveling or camping. Nasal surgery often helps people better tolerate CPAP. The most important thing is not to let obstructive sleep apnea go untreated. It is much cheaper in the long run to treat sleep apnea than to pay for the consequences of not doing so. If you have been unsuccessful in the past, it is now time to reexplore your options. You owe it to your future.

Other Snoring Solutions

If sleep apnea is ruled out and you still snore, physical factors such as a nasal septum deviation might be the culprit, in which case an ear, nose, and throat surgeon can correct the problem and help you breathe better while both asleep and awake, and especially when exercising. Nasal obstruction is common in people with allergies—more about this on the following page.

Many of the same fixes used to treat sleep apnea can also be effective for milder forms of snoring; your doctor may encourage you to lose weight or implement other lifestyle changes such as avoiding alcohol before you go to bed, stopping smoking, or sleeping on your side rather than your back with the aid of a positional therapy device (see opposite). Sleep deprivation can also be a factor in snoring.

Oral appliances, such as those discussed on page 34, are an overlapping therapeutic option for both simple snoring and obstructive sleep apnea. If the level of the obstruction is from the back of the tongue, an oral device may work. If the obstruction is at the level of the nose, however, it won't help the snoring. There are a range of over-the-counter and homeopathic snoring treatments focused on nasal obstruction, including nasal splints, sprays, and drops.

A word of caution about oral devices for snoring, though: Whereas obstructive sleep apnea is a potentially life-threatening condition that is covered by medical insurance, snoring is seen as a cosmetic problem and is not covered. Yet both can be treated with oral appliances. In response, the market is full of inexpensive nonprescription "boil and bite" oral appliances sold as snoring solutions (so named because you customize them yourself by boiling the appliance until it softens and then biting into it to make an impression of your teeth). In truth, these tend to be bulky and ill-fitting (people may spit them out) and are not usually adjustable, leading to potential fixed jaw protrusions. These may also mask the symptoms and delay the treatment of obstructive sleep apnea by simply decreasing snoring without addressing its underlying causes.

Allergies Can Mess Up Your Sleep

Allergies will negatively affect your sleep in many ways. Sleeping with a dog or cat (or any furry animal) can aggravate or trigger pet allergies. Make every effort to keep your pet off your bed and bathe it often—the culprit behind these allergic reactions is most often dander, those dead flakes of skin shed by pets. Chemical allergies can show up when new or unfamiliar detergents are used on our sheets. And since we tend to bury our faces into our pillows, even mild allergies to anything on or inside a pillow can be disruptive. Seasonal allergies can cause nasal obstruction, which can lead to snoring and aggravate any tendencies for sleep apnea. Food allergies will cause babies to have painful reactions and disrupt their sleep (not to mention the rest of the household).

All of these allergy conditions can make you wake feeling tired—as will many allergy medications. If you have known allergies or suddenly suffer from allergic symptoms like sneezing, itchy eyes, or runny nose, discuss with your doctor not only how you feel when you are awake but *also* how it may be affecting your sleep.

THREE

SLEEP FOR THE INSOMNIAC

WHEN I MEET with new patients, I first ask why they've come to see me and what their main concern might be. When they tell me "I can't sleep," my response is "Yes, you can." Everybody sleeps; if you didn't, you'd be dead!

The need for sleep is biological; the way we sleep is learned. Much like learning to eat, we are taught to sleep. All newborn babies drink milk, but five-year-olds around the world have different diets. It's the same with sleep. Even if the origin of your sleep problems is physical, poor sleep lasting a few months or longer almost always has a behavioral component. And once physical barriers to sleep have been dealt with (see Snoring? Start Here, beginning on page 29), the learned behavior is what to focus on.

Ironically, the more logical you are in your approach to sleep, the more likely you are to screw it up. Patients often smile when I tell them this, and you can almost see a light bulb go on over their heads. The right approach to most behavioral sleep problems can be counterintuitive. Many of my patients who are computer engineers in Silicon Valley take a very analytical approach to sleep but end up only messing it up!

In this chapter, I'll help you determine if you're suffering from insomnia and lay out the simple steps you can take to get on a path to a better night's sleep. Although this information is useful for *anyone* who wants to sleep better, insomnia sufferers in particular will benefit from these tips.

Transient versus Chronic Insomnia

When someone who generally sleeps well experiences a night or two of poor sleep, it's often the result of some short-lasting precipitating circumstance—anxiety over the events of the previous day, say, or too much caffeine. (I tend to wake up too early if I have to catch a morning flight, especially when I sleep in hotels.) When these issues resolve, the insomnia disappears. This is known as transient insomnia. In general, this inability to sleep well lasts from one or two nights to one or two weeks. The condition can be repeated intermittently or occur at random, but it is not necessary to consult a physician about it. The danger with transient insomnia is not sleep loss per se but rather the accumulating sleep debt. While doctors are often reluctant to prescribe sleeping pills for stress-induced transient insomnia, the risk/benefit ratio in many instances favors the short-term use of medications. (For more on this, see page 67.)

Insomnia episodes that occur repeatedly need more attention. The problem with chronic insomnia is that its sufferers' sleep becomes unpredictable; they are in a trap. Chronic insomnia can persist for months and even years—the *International Classification of Sleep Disorders* refers to insomnia as "chronic" when it lasts more than three months—and necessitates a completely different approach than that of transient insomnia.

Living with Chronic Insomnia

For people whose sleep is uneventful, it can be difficult to appreciate how insomnia can affect a person's life. After months or years of dealing with unpredictable sleep quality, insomniacs have learned to be hypervigilant about sleep. The thought of sleeping wakes them up! They don't go to bed in a state of serenity, but rather one of uncertainty, wondering how bad their insomnia will be that night. Or they dwell on the past, triggering regrets and uneasiness. Worst of all, they convince themselves that tomorrow will depend on how well they sleep tonight.

Imagine a similar scenario involving eating. Most of us are fortunate enough to be able to more or less predict when and what we will be eating—and that food will always be available if we need it. We can therefore plan our meals based on the assumption that we will be able to eat again in the near future. If you are going out for a big, hearty dinner, for example, you might balance it out with a light lunch that day. But what if your access to food is unpredictable? What if you feel that the quality of food you'll receive is out of your control? What if on some days plenty of good food is available, but on others food is scarce? You might start obsessively stashing food for times of want, and from the moment you wake up until you hit the bed at night, you will be thinking about food. Similarly, when sleep becomes unpredictable, anxiety and hypervigilance understandably result.

Insomnia is often a family affair. Family members—even young children—become sensitized to a loved one's poor sleep habits and will walk on eggshells to avoid disturbing them. When the family makes a good-faith effort to be quiet, and the loved one still has a poor night of sleep, it can pile on more guilt and self-blame—exacerbating an already tenuous situation. In most cases, the insomniac's sleep is not dependent on the behavior of their family but on getting to the root of their own sleep issues.

That said, most insomniacs' sleep problems can improve. Chronic insomnia may have underlying conditions, but it is usually a learned behavior. This is good news, since it is therefore treatable!

Good Sleep Patterns Take Time

It's understandable: You want to sleep so desperately that you're impatient, eager for quick fixes. But you're not going to change years of poor sleep in just a few days. These are ingrained patterns that are resistant to disruption—and often we want to sleep so badly we give up before we can solidify new habits. If you decide whether or not a new strategy is working based on a night or two of trying, you can end up further aggravating your sleep hypervigilance and insomnia.

To make sleep changes truly stick, strive to practice the techniques laid out in this chapter for six to eight weeks. Expect to feel new sleep habits take hold after a couple of weeks, followed by steady, noticeable improvement. It's normal to be frustrated or unsettled at first, but be patient—remember that the brain is quick to pick up on your frustrations. If your brain thinks something is wrong, it will avoid sleeping or will sleep only in short spurts.

While you're applying these rules to your sleep, it's a good idea to keep a sleep diary to track the amount of time you're in bed. You'll also want to record what kind of day you're having: Are you feeling refreshed, alert? Or are you feeling fatigued, listless, irritable? By reviewing your notes, you can track your sleep improvements over time.

Insomnia Is a Thinker's Condition

Consider a typical day. If you accomplished eight things out of ten on that day's to-do list, you had a really good day. As soon as you hit the sack, however, the two things you *failed* to do float up into your mind. Now you want to sleep but also don't want to forget what needs to be done. This is counterproductive. We are all amnestic as we fall asleep. (You may be able to tell me what time you went to bed, but you cannot tell me what time you fell asleep!) It's far better to set up a scheduled thinking time prior to bedtime, to help get this worry out of your system well before you need to sleep.

Most people are never alone with their thoughts until they hop into bed, when the day's distractions fall away. This is why they have trouble "turning off" their brains or insist they must have a television or radio on in the background to block their thoughts with distractions until they drift off to sleep. While it's true that the brain never actually turns off, there are effective techniques to keep racing or recurring thoughts from disturbing your sleep.

Simply reserve some time away from the bedroom for approximately fifteen to thirty minutes every night, preferably after all work and activities are finished. Sit in a quiet place, away from the bedroom, with a paper notebook—not a laptop or phone (see page 71)—and write down whatever you need to accomplish tomorrow. Start with writing down mundane tasks such as chores. Then list those things you've been meaning to do but haven't gotten around to, like sending a thank-you for a birthday gift or calling an old friend. Include anything that is worrying you or on your mind. Finally, jot down those things you have always wanted to do or places you've wanted to go. Give yourself some time to be alone with these thoughts, then close the notebook and tell yourself, "I am done with my day; whatever is not done can wait till tomorrow." *Say it and believe it.* Then spend some time doing something relaxing, such as reading for pleasure or taking a bath. Think of it as a reward for having finished your day. When you feel those yawns coming on and start getting drowsy, climb into bed.

If your mind starts to race again, remind yourself that the important stuff is already written down, the day is over, and you are prepared for tomorrow. In the morning when you wake up, take a moment to reread what you wrote the previous night. You'll find that the problems you were so worried about often seem less burdensome in the morning light. Continue with scheduled thinking time every night as a routine. If you're like most of my patients, your tendency to wake up with racing thoughts during the night will diminish.

Escape the Worry Trap

Worrying about sleep can be a trap. If you go to bed thinking that tomorrow's success depends on how well you sleep tonight, you are setting yourself up for a troubled night of sleep. Worry sends a warning signal to the brain, which responds by staying alert and sleeping as little as possible. Your brain is just doing what it is supposed to do: Sleeping is one of our most potentially dangerous activities—it's when we are at our most vulnerable. Your brain interprets danger and stress as the same thing and sleeping lightly or not at all is its biological response to an alert that something is wrong.

At the same time, sleep is a homeostatic function of the brain. Homeostasis is the mechanism that a biological system uses to achieve balance. This means that our brain strives to restore itself during sleep. It is a simple yet powerful concept. Don't be hard on yourself if you wake up during the night; remember, waking frequently is a normal function of a sleep cycle (see page 18). Trying to stop this process only sets in motion an endless vicious cycle of waking fitfully and sleeping in spurts. Comfort yourself by knowing that sleep will return. The brain's homeostatic drive guarantees it.

THE HYPERVIGILANCE OF AN INSOMNIAC

My longtime patient Judith was a gruff New Yorker and proud of it. She smoked cigarettes, gambled, and didn't mind a cocktail. If she didn't like you, she would let you know it—though she would reveal her sweet, kind side once you gained her respect and trust. I was thirty-two years old when she first started seeing me, and she referred to me as "the kid." She did not do well with CBT-I (see page 54), and we shared many ups and downs in finding the right treatment for her insomnia.

Judith had been taking zolpidem (aka Ambien) in a 10 mg dose with moderate success—she was still having trouble sleeping. When a new formulation of zolpidem with an increased dosage of 12.5 mg came on the market, she asked if she could try it. I gave her some professional samples and told her to let me know how it worked.

The following morning, I received an urgent message from a pharmacist, who had an upset customer. Judith had arrived at the pharmacy when it opened, convinced she'd received a placebo because the 12.5 mg formulation had done nothing at all for her, and she'd stayed up all night fretting about not getting her sleep. Judith had asked the pharmacist to show her what the new 12.5 mg tablet looked like. When I called Judith to reassure her the samples were real, she said, "Lucky for you, what you gave me matches what the pharmacy has!"

As I listened to my patient, I thought about the hyper-vigilance of sleep in people with insomnia. I gathered that her suspicions that I was trying to trick her with a placebo made her upset, which kept her from sleeping. The novelty of simply changing a dose of medication had heightened her hypervigilance. A change that should have improved her sleep briefly exacerbated her insomnia. I told her to keep taking the medication for the next couple of nights. At the end of the week, she called and said she was sleeping better, and she continued taking the 12.5 mg dosage.

On any given day, you may or may not sleep well. If you are making a change to your sleep routine, stick with it for several days before you decide if something is helpful or not. In making judgments on the efficacy of a new treatment based on one night, you can end up chasing your tail and further aggravate your sleep hypervigilance and insomnia.

THE WORRY TRAP: CASE STUDY 2

INSOMNIA AND THE PLACEBO EFFECT

If you look at the prescribing information for any sleeping pill, you'll see a comparison of the side effects of those who took the medication and those who received a placebo. That's right, the placebo group often reports side effects! A common example is next-day sedation, or a sleep hangover.

Why would a placebo have side effects? Put yourself in the place of an insomniac participating in the research trial of a new medication. You've volunteered because you hope the new medication will help you finally sleep better. Volunteers for such a trial are usually asked to stop taking any sleep aids, and so one's insomnia may worsen for a short time as a result. Once the trial starts, it's natural to assume you've lucked out and gotten the new active agent and not the placebo. As a result, your hypervigilance may be lowered. Mix this lower hypervigilance with a buildup of several nights of poor sleep, and you—along with many other people in the placebo group—will report better sleep. Because you're likely sleeping longer than usual, you may wake up feeling groggy (more on this on page 24). But instead of realizing this is a normal reaction, you report next-day sedation as a side effect of the new medication!

Because catching up on sleep can make us feel groggy, I routinely warn my patients to avoid reaching conclusions after only one night of taking a new medication.

Lock In a Wake-up Time

People with insomnia often focus on their difficulty falling asleep and are able to provide loads of details about their bedtime, the time it took them to drift off, how often they woke up, and how long they were awake during the night. But when asked about their wake-up time, the answer becomes vague—"it depends," they say, "on when I fell asleep." One of the first steps in fixing a behavioral component of a sleep problem is to lock in a wake-up time. Patients with insomnia often say they will do "anything" to sleep better, but when I ask them to get out of the bed at the same time every day their first response is "I can't do that." But the fact is, it is much easier to force yourself to wake up at a specific time than to fall asleep. If you wake up and get out of bed at the same time every day, eventually your robust biological clock will also help make the time at which you fall asleep more predictable.

Increase Your Sleep Gradually

Increasing your total sleep time in a single night is hard to do. Blame the conflict between the homeostatic drive for sleep and the circadian fluctuation in the sleep/wake schedule. These two physiological systems can oppose each other. Your homeostatic system may want you to sleep longer, while your circadian system—anticipating that "dawn" will occur about the same time that it occurred the previous morning—wakes you before you get the additional sleep you crave.

If you are trying to increase your average daily sleep time by one hour, introduce your new habits gradually: For a week or two, go to bed only fifteen minutes earlier than usual and get out of bed fifteen minutes later than usual. If you find yourself falling asleep easily and waking up on time, repeat the process, going to bed fifteen minutes earlier and waking up fifteen minutes later. Extending your sleep by thirty minutes, getting used to this new routine, then adding another thirty minutes is an easier way of accomplishing your goal of extending total sleep time by an hour.

Hacks for Getting Back to Sleep

Many people with insomnia spend more time in bed awake than sleeping—and no longer associate the bed with sleep. The more the bed is used for activities other than sleep, the weaker the connection will be between bed and sleep. Let this be your mantra: *The bedroom is for sleeping.*

If you wake during the night and have trouble getting back to sleep, employ these strategies:

- **Don't look at the clock.** Turn your alarm facing away from you, if you must. If you want to know what time it is, it's nighttime, that's what time it is!

- **Lie calmly and focus on your breathing.** Reassure yourself that sleep will come. It always does.

- **If after a few minutes you find yourself getting restless, get up and leave your bedroom.** Don't do anything productive such as chores or work (this will serve as a positive reinforcement of your difficulty staying asleep). Read something of no value—your refrigerator warranty, for example.

- **Don't turn on the computer or TV.** Finding something interesting to read or watch will only make things worse by rewarding the insomnia and the vicious cycle it perpetuates. Again, pick up that refrigerator warranty!

- **Don't grab a snack.** Eating can also be a reward, reinforcing your insomnia (not to mention that late-night eating correlates to weight gain).

- **Keep reminding yourself that your sleepiness will eventually return.** When that happens, get back in bed—not on a couch or chair.

You *Don't* Want to Sleep like a Baby . . .

It is a misconception that infancy is the best sleep time of our lives. The reality is that babies sleep only for brief periods, with sleep cycles regularly interrupted by a need to feed every two to four hours during the night. (Babies do sleep deeply when they go down, however, and are able to snooze through just about any loud noise. If you find yourself tiptoeing around at naptime, afraid of waking the baby, relax—baby is deep in dreamland.)

. . . You *Do* Want to Sleep like a Nine-Year-Old

The best sleepers in our society? Children in elementary school. Consider the lifestyle of a typically healthy and happy second or third grader: They come home from school, have a snack, do a little homework. Dinner and play follow, but a set bedtime is the house rule—and parents still tend to tuck them in and even read them to sleep. When you are nine years old, you don't need to worry about the rent or mortgage. You are woken up, given breakfast, and delivered to school. Nine-year-olds tend to fall asleep easily, appear to sleep through the night, and wake up refreshed. During the day, they are full of energy and don't nap.

These children have a consistent routine, and they fall asleep in a state of serenity, feeling safe, comfortable, and loved. It's how we should all sleep. So if you are having trouble falling and/or staying asleep, don't be hard on yourself. You'll sleep better if you go to bed in the right frame of mind. No matter how much stress you are under when you are awake, you will sleep better if you reframe your mindset, give yourself a little love and positive reinforcement, and tuck yourself in. Your life is a reflection of how you sleep, and how you sleep is a reflection of your life.

Distinguish between Being Tired and Sleepy

Many people complain of feeling tired but frustrated that they cannot fall asleep, or even go out of their way to make themselves *more* tired in a seemingly fruitless attempt to fall asleep. If you got up and did one hundred jumping jacks, you might feel tired, but it's likely you won't feel sleepy. (Evening exercise can actually rev you up—see page 58 for more on sleep and exercise.)

The terms tired and sleepy actually mean two different things. This is a simple but important distinction. You could spend a full week in a luxury hotel room doing nothing at all. You won't feel tired, but you will periodically sleep. Low thyroid hormone levels can also make you feel tired but not sleepy. Make a point in distinguishing sheer fatigue from sleepiness, because each requires a different solution. If you are tired, you need to rest, and if you are sleepy, you need to sleep.

Think of Napping like Snacking

If you skimped on eating a full meal, having a snack between meals is okay. But if snacking keeps you from eating when dinnertime comes around, then the habit has become a problem. It's the same with sleep: Napping can decrease your appetite for sleep and hinder your ability to get a full night's sleep—but it can also satisfy the sleep hunger of the sleep deprived. (In fact, if you start having vivid dreams during a very short nap, that's a sure sign you are sleep deprived.)

Ideally, naps should be brief. Somewhere around forty minutes should satisfy. Longer naps, especially more than ninety minutes, can make you feel sluggish when you awaken. This phenomenon is sometimes called sleep drunkenness and is attributed to a physiological process called sleep inertia. In essence, once we sleep that long, we want to *keep* sleeping, so we wake up feeling out of sorts.

A short nap during the day, however, can do wonders to energize you—which is why the idea of napping in the workplace is undergoing a cultural shift. Why is eating lunch at your desk viewed as a sign of dedication to your work but taking a nap at your desk considered lazy? Well-rested employees lead to increased productivity, a fact that has led some workplaces to introduce fancy napping pods, nap rooms, and other innovations.

I bet if you had a quick lunch and took a twenty-minute power nap during the rest of your break time, you'd finish the day a more alert, productive, and happy employee!

Some people with insomnia tell me they fall asleep in a recliner or sofa after lunch, then can't fall asleep in their own beds at night. If this happens to you, try to nap in the same place you sleep at night. It's further reinforcement that bed is the place for sleeping.

CBT-I for Good Sleep

If the preceding strategies were not sufficient to relieve your insomnia, then cognitive behavioral therapy for insomnia (CBT-I) may be the right solution for you. CBT-I has an impressive success rate in treating insomnia: More than two-thirds of people with chronic insomnia who undergo CBT-I are able to sleep better without relying on medications in about two months. (If that sounds like a long time, consider that for people who have endured years of poor sleep, two months is a worthy investment for a lifetime of sleeping well!)

CBT-I can be done in group settings, or one-on-one with a therapist. People with milder forms of insomnia may find they can apply CBT-I principles on their own and improve their sleep (there are apps available online).

CBT-I is based on the assumption that chronic insomniacs sleep a certain way because of past bad sleep experiences and misconceptions, which have led them to develop sleep behaviors they believe are necessary but can instead exacerbate their problem. When you suffer from insomnia, sleep becomes a fascinating subject. Your family members and friends give you unsolicited sleep advice. You read about sleep more than most people and naturally assume you know a whole lot about sleep. But when using CBT-I therapies, you may find that a piece of information you swear by has set you off down the wrong path. For example, you may initially sleep better after drinking alcohol, but drinking nightly will only make sleep issues worse in the long term.

The goal of CBT-I is to give you information to help you think differently about sleep and to make behavioral adjustments that result in incremental improvements. These improvements inspire further changes in your thinking and behavior, and gradually, the process snowballs to reverse the vicious cycle of insomnia.

One of the most frustrating things about insomnia is the feeling that you are wasting hours trying to get to sleep. You might spend eight hours in bed but sleep only five. This wasted time trying to sleep may make you feel that sleep is out of your control. Sleep restriction, a common CBT-I behavioral technique, dictates a narrower window of time that you actually spend in bed, typically five and a half to seven hours, with a fixed wake-up time (regardless of how well you slept the night before). Sleep is avoided at any other time of the day. Under sleep restriction, the body's homeostatic drive improves the ability to stay asleep. As sleep improves, you gradually increase the time in bed (short intervals of fifteen to thirty minutes about once a week) until you are satisfied with the amount of sleep you are getting.

As you work through this sleep restriction process, you might apply stimulus control as well. Typical stimulus control instructions are designed to reinforce the connection between the bedroom and sleep, and include going to bed only when you are sleepy and getting out of bed when you cannot sleep. If you are tossing and turning in bed and only getting frustrated, there are additional steps you can take to get your sleep back on track: see Hacks for Getting Back to Sleep, page 50.

Along with sleep restriction and stimulus control, you can also incorporate relaxation exercises or mindfulness meditation (such as the ones discussed on page 59) to help lower any anxiety you may have about sleeping. The aim is to push away ruminating, worried thoughts about your sleep. One of my favorite techniques to help stem these ruminating thoughts is scheduled thinking time (see page 43).

FOUR

A DAY IN THE (NIGHT) LIFE

JUST AS THE quality of our sleep affects our waking life, how we behave during the day plays a role in our sleep. This chapter addresses the myriad effects of food and drink, exercise, electronic devices, medications, bedding, and more on sleep. It also explores how integrating certain behaviors, like meditation or relaxation techniques, into your daily routine can help promote sleep. Finally, it addresses some of the most common sleep issues we face as we move through the world, from tricks for sleeping on planes to how to adjust to daylight saving time.

ACTIVITY

Exercise and Sleep

Regular physical exercise—even as little as ten minutes a day—helps people fall asleep faster, increases total sleep time, and improves overall sleep quality. Physical activity increases the secretion of human growth hormone (HGH), which promotes restorative, deeper sleep. Overall fitness helps keep weight down and improves your mood, which also lead to healthier sleep. Exercise bolsters sleep in other ways, too, such as by reducing stress.

But the scientific community has yet to reach a consensus on the best *time* to exercise for optimal sleep. Because it takes a while for the adrenaline and heat generated by a workout to dissipate, brisk exercise right before bedtime can backfire. When I first entered the sleep field, the teaching was that evening exercise may make it harder to fall asleep and stay asleep. Yet, for many people, evening is probably the most convenient time to exercise—we are usually in a rush to get to school or work in the morning, and exercising during the middle of the workday can be impractical. For a long time, my advice to patients having trouble sleeping was to limit themselves to passive stretching or peaceful yoga exercises in the evening. However, more recent studies have found that the timing of exercise may not really matter. Evening exercise can make it harder to fall asleep, but once some people fall asleep, their sleep itself is deeper. Doing vigorous exercise within an hour of bedtime still has the potential to disrupt sleep, so get your routine in well before you hit the sack. But don't use the time of day as an excuse not to exercise.

Meditation for Mindful Sleep

It has been said that sleep is the best meditation. But many folks who have trouble sleeping turn to meditation for help in quieting a busy mind. As mentioned on page 56, mindfulness meditation techniques and breathing exercises are often incorporated into behavioral therapies to treat insomnia. It makes sense: People with insomnia are prone to racing thoughts and excessive rumination about the potential catastrophic consequences of not being able to sleep. Mindfulness techniques train our minds to stay in the moment and not wander off on self-defeating tangents of regret and worry.

You can practice meditation anywhere and anytime, but for poor sleepers it's best to start in a quiet, calming environment, right before you go to bed. Close your eyes and focus on steady, deep, natural breathing. You can visualize a relaxing scene (a beach or fluffy clouds) or place your hand on your belly and focus on the rising and falling of your breath. Or imagine your breath slowly making its way up from your toes to your head every time you inhale. There are many apps available that offer guided meditations, including some specifically focused on sleeping.

Know that it's common for the mind to wander at first, so don't get frustrated; gently direct your focus back to meditative breathing. Try to commit to meditating for ten minutes a day for at least eight weeks before you decide it's not helpful.

Does Sex Make People Sleepy?

Whenever I'm asked this question, I turn it around and ask the questioners about *their* experiences with sleep and sex. Sexuality is so highly variable that it's not surprising that I get a wide range of responses. You might think that having sex would promote sleep (and it can), but humans can have sex any time of the day. If we abruptly fell asleep anytime we made love, that would be inconvenient, to say the least! In general, having an orgasm *can* help you feel sleepy if you are already in the mood to sleep (an orgasm releases prolactin, which promotes sleepiness and relaxation, along with oxytocin, which promotes calmness and social bonding). But given the physical exertion and flood of chemical changes, sex makes others feel energized.

FOOD AND DRINK

Alcohol Is a Double-Edged Sword

Drinking alcohol will help you fall asleep faster. If you drink enough of it, it can even make you pass out. But it won't help you stay asleep. Alcohol disrupts the natural restorative effect of sleep and is metabolized too quickly to provide a full night's sleep. Because alcohol is a sedative, the sleep you get is more akin to feeling knocked out than sleeping restfully. Even worse, alcohol can exacerbate serious sleep conditions like obstructive sleep apnea.

A number of over-the-counter nighttime sleep aids rely on a combination of alcohol and antihistamines. The alcohol helps initiate sleep quickly and the antihistamine helps a person maintain sleep. However, the efficacy of these products wears off quickly—after a few days—and they become unreliable. More important, they do not address the core reasons someone is having trouble sleeping in the first place.

Caffeine Is Complicated

Given the epidemic levels of sleep deprivation in our society, it's not surprising that coffee bars are booming. Caffeine is the most widely consumed psychostimulant worldwide, with 90 percent of adults reporting regular caffeine use. I, like most doctors, generally advocate one of the old sleep hygiene rules: avoiding caffeine six to eight hours before bed. But new research on how caffeine is metabolized by our bodies and how it affects our brains tells us that the old rules are not that simple anymore.

In moderation, caffeine has generally been shown to lead to increased health and quality of life. General guidelines for caffeine consumption advise adults to limit their caffeine intake to between 200 mg and 400 mg per day, about two to four regular cups of coffee. Not everyone responds to caffeine the same way, however. Caffeine's effects depend on many factors, including individual genetic traits for metabolism, as well as age, liver disease, obesity, smoking history, and diet. Caffeine also interacts with many medications. For example, the use of oral contraceptives increases caffeine's half-life (meaning its effects are prolonged). Some individuals are hypersensitive to the effects of caffeine, while about of the population is relatively caffeine resistant, or hyposensitive. Repeated exposure to caffeine can lead to higher tolerance of its side effects. Ultimately, listen to your own body. If you see no ill effects from your after-dinner cup, enjoy!

All that being said, bragging that you can drink coffee before going to bed and still fall asleep is not something to be proud of. Our brains run on a molecule called adenosine triphosphate (ATP). As our ATP is depleted, a by-product called adenosine builds in our brains. The higher the adenosine levels in our brains, the sleepier we feel. Caffeine blocks our brains' adenosine receptor, which is why it makes us feel less sleepy. So if you can fall asleep after a shot of espresso, it may mean that you have built up so much adenosine in your brain from sleep debt (see page 23) that coffee is not sufficient to keep you awake.

Water Is Not a Problem, Until It Is

Normally when we are sleeping, our bodies produce less urine, so we can sleep longer without interruption. Many people go to sleep with a glass of water at their bedside, particularly in winter, when heating systems can be drying, or if they've eaten a salty or spicy evening meal—this is totally fine. If you need a glass of water at your bedside because you routinely wake up with a dry mouth, however, you are likely snoring and mouth breathing and should see your doctor. Some medications can also make you feel thirsty.

If you consistently wake up thirsty *and* needing to urinate, you may have sleep apnea and should contact your health-care provider (see page 136). This is especially likely if you also snore or wake up unrefreshed. Having to wake up to get rid of fluid at the same time you need a drink of water means something may be wrong with the biology of your sleep. When there is a narrowing in the throat, such as in obstructive sleep apnea, a cascade of events occurs that culminates in the kidneys making *more* urine, not less. If the signal to empty your bladder is strong enough, you wake up to urinate. If you sleep through the signal, you will wet the bed. (This is why it's usually a mistake to restrict water from a child who is bed-wetting. Simply drinking water is not usually the cause of a child's bed-wetting; other physical factors play a much bigger role. For more on bed-wetting, see page 115.)

Don't Eat Two Hours Prior to Bedtime

Eating close to bedtime can be problematic for several reasons. Having a full stomach in bed can exacerbate acid reflux and lead to heartburn, a real sleep disturber (see next page). And while it's a common misconception that eating foods high in sugar before bed will make us hyper and interfere with our sleep (that's not how the brain handles sugar), what *is* true is that late-night consumption of any food is more likely to make us gain weight. It's even got a name—nocturnal eating syndrome—which is associated with obesity. When we're tired and sleep deprived, we're often more impulsive in our food choices and may eat rich, fatty, or otherwise unhealthy things that we usually avoid. It is easy to mindlessly eat when we are sleepy or want to stay awake when we should be asleep. Finally, some medications taken at night work better on an empty stomach. Food can affect the absorption of medications such as sleeping pills, leading to fluctuating results or compromised efficacy.

On the other hand, don't make a habit of going to bed hungry—it can disrupt sleep, break down muscle mass, and even reinforce eating disorders around sleep.

Heartburn and Sleep

Heartburn is a symptom of gastroesophageal reflux disease (GERD), a condition caused by stomach acid moving upward into the esophagus. A valve made of muscle at the junction of the esophagus and stomach allows food to enter the stomach and prevents the stomach contents from coming back up the esophagus. But when this valve malfunctions, the result is acid damage. GERD is more common during pregnancy and just one more reason women sleep poorly at this time (for more on sleep and pregnancy, see page 120). For most people, infrequent heartburn is not a serious problem. If persistent, however, heartburn can lead to medical complications, including significant damage to the esophagus and a higher risk of esophageal cancer.

Ways to treat heartburn range from medication to surgery to recognizing the common triggers and minimizing them. Gravity seems to play a role, since lying down can cause acidic contents to come up, and many people who suffer from heartburn feel the effects most acutely at bedtime. Sometimes the reflux can be so bad you may awaken with a bitter taste in your mouth. A common strategy to lower the symptoms of GERD is to avoid sleeping flat—by adding pillows to raise the upper half of your body, for example. Decreasing caffeine intake, eating smaller meals, avoiding alcohol close to bedtime, and quitting smoking are also helpful. An overlooked factor for reflux in some people is obstructive sleep apnea (see page 31). The reflux can affect your sleep, and the sleep apnea can make GERD worse. Get your sleep apnea treated, and any GERD symptoms are likely to improve.

Warm Milk for Better Sleep?

In some households, a traditional nighttime ritual is to offer children a glass of warm milk before tucking them into bed. It likely originated as an extension of nighttime nursing for younger children, who historically were breastfed longer than is common now. A glass of warm milk at bedtime may relax adults who retain pleasant memories of this loving childhood tradition. It's also a nice protein-packed snack to prevent you from going to bed with an empty stomach. The warm milk itself contains no chemical properties that promote sleep or help a person with insomnia sleep better. But if you enjoy the tradition, there is no reason to stop it.

Herbal Tea for Bedtime

There are many different teas marketed to help you sleep. Any of these can promote sleep if used occasionally. Blends to help you sleep typically include valerian and chamomile; chamomile alone does not consistently aid sleep, but valerian has a mild sedative effect and can make you drowsy when you first take it. These sedating properties eventually wear off with nightly use, however, especially if the underlying reason for difficulty sleeping is not addressed. For a person suffering from chronic insomnia, no herbal tea alone is sufficient to remedy the situation. Still, there's nothing wrong with using tea as a part of a relaxing routine at the end of the day.

Sleep Claims Are Fishy When It Comes to Seafood (and Poultry)

Scattered reports that eating seafood helps people sleep better are not backed by science. Studies reveal that the amount of improvement from eating seafood is relatively small; in general, subjects did not report much better sleep compared with people taking the placebo. For some folks, nutrients such as zinc and vitamin B_6 in fish may have some positive effects. But if you have a significant problem with insomnia, becoming a pescatarian is not likely to solve the issue.

On the subject of food and sleep, it's a myth that eating large amounts of the amino acid tryptophan, found in turkey and chicken, will make you sleepy. In controlled studies, people consuming large amounts of tryptophan were not any sleepier than those in the placebo group. Yes, you may feel sleepy after a large Thanksgiving meal, but blame overeating, weariness from traveling, dining in the afternoon (when our alert levels dip), drinking alcohol with the meal, or simply being in a relaxed state while off from work for making you feel groggy post-turkey.

SLEEPING PILLS, MEDICATIONS, AND SUPPLEMENTS

The State of Sleeping Pills

Prescription sleeping pills (also known as hypnotics) are now definitely safer in some ways than they were in the past, when heavy-duty barbiturates and quaaludes were prescribed for sleep. These days, the trend is for prescription sleeping pills to be safer rather than stronger. In fact, some over-the-counter sleeping aids can cause more dangerous overdose reactions than current prescription sleeping pills. Occasionally using a hypnotic to help you fight off temporary insomnia (when your mother-in-law comes to visit, say) is okay.

But for a person who has had trouble falling and/or staying asleep for more than three months (a condition called chronic insomnia—see page 40), nighttime becomes a period of fretful uncertainty. Bringing sleeping pills into the mix can add another layer of worry, especially if relief is palpable. *How bad will it be tonight?* the insomniac may wonder. *Will I need one pill or two? What if I run out of pills?* When people report that they can't sleep without their prescription sleeping pill, its usage has become a problem. One of the main reasons sleeping pills require prescriptions is that they can be habit forming. The overall goal of any sleep medication is that the patient sleeps easily throughout the night and wakes up refreshed *without* relying on medication. Most people with insomnia sleep better when the root cause of their insomnia is addressed—see Sleep for the Insomniac, beginning on page 39.

Skip "Natural" Sleep Aids for More Natural Sleep

Health food store shelves are lined with "natural" sleep aids. Many have a mildly sedating effect that usually diminishes over time. But being sedated is not the same as naturally sleeping. In general, these aids are best used for the occasional bout of insomnia; when it comes to chronic insomnia, many sleep aids that seem to work at first eventually lose efficacy. In the long run, relying on supplements does not address the underlying causes for poor sleep. Here's a rundown of the most popular supplements on the market.

- **Cannabidiol (CBD).** There is growing interest in the use of the cannabis derivative CBD for many therapeutic applications, and sleep is one of them. In fact, preliminary research and a growing number of anecdotal reports show that CBD may actually be helpful in the treatment of insomnia. But until randomized long-term clinical trials are completed, it's hard to recommend CBD. We need to see if benefits are sustained, and if there is any downside.

- **GABA, or gamma-aminobutyric acid,** is an amino acid and one of the most important neurotransmitters in the brain. It helps reduce anxiety and promote sleep. Many common prescription sleeping pills (such as Ambien) work by increasing the activity of GABA in our brains. This naturally occurring chemical is also sold in over-the-counter supplements; when GABA is digested by your stomach, however, it is unlikely to have much of an effect on your brain and cannot reliably make you very sleepy.

- **Magnesium** has a calming effect; milk of magnesium used as a laxative works to relax our intestinal muscles. But the evidence that magnesium supplements help with chronic insomnia is not strong.

- **Melatonin** is a naturally occurring hormone released by the pineal gland in the brain in anticipation of the evening. Melatonin supplements may help adults fall asleep faster (and studies show it *does* help children fall asleep faster), but it does not aid in staying asleep or significantly increasing the total sleep time in most people. The purity and quality of various melatonin preparations fluctuate widely—what is labeled on the bottle is often very different from what is in the actual pills. This fluctuation may be a reason that reactions to it vary, with some folks saying melatonin doesn't work and others claiming it knocks them out.

Some Medications May Be Making Your Insomnia Worse

Many medications can adversely affect your sleep, and you may not even know it. Propranolol, a commonly prescribed medication for blood pressure control and migraine prevention, can cause insomnia, as can oral steroids such as prednisone. Many over-the-counter cold and allergy medications have sedating effects, but others are intended for daytime use—taking daytime cold meds at night can alter your sleep. And a number of over-the-counter preparations contain caffeine, including common analgesics and pain relievers.

Prescription drugs come with a complete list of side effects and contraindications; if you develop insomnia after starting or changing a medication, tell your pharmacist or prescriber about it. If you suspect that your sleep is being disturbed by a medication, always check with your prescribing health-care provider before you stop taking it, since abruptly stopping some medications can be unsafe.

It's important to consider not only the type of medication you take but the time you take it. This is especially true for controlled-release formulations of medications used to treat attention deficit disorder. Controlled-release medications are designed to provide a longer duration of action, which can disrupt sleep. To counter the effects of the medication, you might then be prescribed a sleeping aid—which results in what's known as a polypharmacy situation, piling medications upon medications. Talk to your practitioner about the best times to take controlled-release formulations to avoid sleep disruptions.

Antidepressants are another case where timing can be important: Some are sedating, while others have alerting effects, and switching between antidepressants is fairly common for long-term patients. If your doctor switched your sedating antidepressant for one with stimulative properties, and out of habit you take it at night, it may be the reason you aren't sleeping well.

DEVICES AND TECHNOLOGY

The Blue-Light Effect

Blue color light frequencies play a special role in our body's circadian clock and our sleep schedule. A type of photoreceptor in our eyes, called intrinsically photosensitive retinal ganglion cells, preferentially react to light in the blue spectrum to help regulate our circadian rhythms. Once it was understood that these special neurons preferentially react to blue light, the idea of blocking out the blue-light frequencies coming off of our screens became popular, because it theoretically allows us to use these devices late at night without causing significant shifts in the circadian system.

Blue-light filtering strategies do work to decrease the effects of light on delaying our circadian clock, but the blue-light frequencies are not the only reason electronic devices keep us up at night. Our engagement with the devices and their content likely plays a much bigger role. Using blue-light blockers is like putting a filter on a cigarette. Yes, it can help, but it doesn't address the core problem.

Wearables Are Just Tools

Portable devices to measure sleep have been available for decades in the clinical and scientific setting, but with the advent of smartphones and wearable devices, the technology has become much more widely available. And clearly, judging by the rapid growth in the popularity of sleep trackers and wearable devices, the public is recognizing the importance of sleep more than ever. I don't discourage patients from using these devices; I'm glad when someone values their sleep. But I'm not sure what information people are really looking to get out of them. You don't monitor your refrigerator with a separate temperature control to make sure it's working properly. If the food is cold in the morning, you trust that the fridge was running during the night. In the same way, if you wake up feeling refreshed in the morning and are energetic throughout the day, then you are unlikely to need a sleep tracker. Conversely, knowing you slept poorly doesn't do anything to help you *not* sleep poorly again the next night.

Wearable sleep-tracking devices may be of value if you have a change in your prior pattern of sleep, which might indicate that something else in your body is changing, too. But obsessing over the results from these devices can be problematic. Different devices can give very different results in the same person on the same night. *Orthosomnia* is a term that has even been coined to describe people who develop worsening sleep issues from using these devices in a quest for sleep perfection! Get a wearable if you're curious—just don't lose sleep worrying about the results.

White Noise: A Sonic Lullaby

Although every noise that occurs while we're sleeping has the potential to rouse us, it's those that are significantly louder than the usual background sounds that generally wake us up. The reason is not so much the noise itself but the sudden shift in our sonic environment. Abrupt noises like a smoke alarm going off have a purpose: to wake and alert. But if honking horns, loud neighbors, or a clunky furnace are interrupting your sleep, what can you do?

White noise is a machine-generated sound designed to mask these disruptive sonic shifts and provide a consistent, pleasing sound throughout the night. White-noise machines work by introducing a uniform background noise to our environment that we become accustomed to and associate with sleep. By raising the volume of a familiar sound, we are less likely to notice a sudden unwanted noise.

A white-noise machine is a useful tool for anyone who sleeps in an unpleasantly noisy environment, especially if the noise is intermittent or unpredictable. Many people travel with their white-noise machines, to help them sleep in unfamiliar beds. Some people even use white-noise machines when they are sleeping in an environment that is too *quiet* for their liking. Pets have been shown to benefit from sleeping with white noise, too, as a soothing antidote to separation anxiety.

Some white-noise machines play only one tone, while others have all sorts of comforting tracks, from nature sounds like rain or ocean surf to ambient noises like whirring fans. Inexpensive white-noise apps can also work, but many of these devices use recordings that loop and repeat, which can disturb a person who is hypervigilant to noise and looping repetition.

White noise is not the only game in town. While white-noise sound includes all frequencies audible to the human ear at the same volume, other types of machines filter out only certain frequencies. Pink noise has some higher frequencies filtered out, so it sounds more like rain. Brown noise has even more high frequencies filtered out, giving it more of a low-tone rumble. In the end, it's all about personal preference. When you find one that works for you, it can be a lifetime comfort.

Earplugs for Sleeping

I have mixed feelings about the use of earplugs during sleep. Yes, they help block noise and are incredibly easy to use. And they work fine as a temporary solution to an unusual and noisy sleeping situation, like when staying somewhere other than your own home. When a person believes earplugs are essential to their sleep, however, it's a problem.

People with insomnia suffer from unpredictable sleep quality. If on a given night they use earplugs and get a solid night of sleep, they suddenly become hypervigilant around noise. Now, because they are going to sleep believing they must be vigilant about noises to help themselves sleep, their brain forces them to sleep more lightly. In time, they do sleep more lightly, and the earplugs stop being effective.

THE BEDROOM ENVIRONMENT

The Bed as a Place for Sleeping

Using the bed only for sleeping is part of the standard sleep hygiene rules. The idea being that if you use the bed for other activities such as reading or watching TV, your body will get used to being awake in bed. For sufferers of chronic insomnia, it is worth following the Hacks for Getting Back to Sleep described starting on page 50 to help reinforce the connection between bed and sleep.

That said, I often meet people who tell me they like to read in bed but feel guilty about it because it's "bad." Well, it *is* bad—if you struggle to sleep at night. If you sleep well, you can do whatever you like in bed! I compare it with eating chocolate cake for breakfast. If you suffer from diabetes, it's not a good idea, but if you are otherwise healthy, it's a nice occasional treat.

Most Like It Cool

We tend to sleep best in cooler environments, because a drop in our body temperature usually makes us feel sleepy. Although preferences depend on the individual, keeping the bedroom temperature between 60 and 70 degrees Fahrenheit (15.5 to 21 degrees Celsius) should help facilitate sleep.

One of the unexplained aspects of sleep is that while we are typically able to maintain an average core body temperature of 98.6 degrees Fahrenheit (37 degrees Celsius), this regulation of our core temperature decreases when we are in REM sleep, a phenomenon called poikilothermy. Since REM dominates the last third of the night (as discussed on page 16), this may be why in the beginning of the night we kick off our covers, but in the early-morning hours we are fighting over the blankets with our bed partner.

Night Light

As discussed on page 71, light has a tremendous influence on our circadian rhythms, which makes it essential to control how much light we are exposed to in the hours immediately prior to and during sleeping. Experiencing artificial light at night can trick our brains into behaving as if it is a short summer night, causing us to go to sleep later. If you're having trouble sleeping, start gradually limiting your exposure to light sources about two hours before bedtime; leave electronic devices out of the bedroom and turn any lighted clocks away from sight lines. Blackout blinds and eye masks can further block unwanted light.

It's Probably Not the Mattress

Typically, insomniacs sleep better away from home because they associate their own bedrooms with places of frustration and lack of shut-eye. This may be why many people sleep better when staying at a hotel. They may (inaccurately) attribute their improved sleep to the change in mattress instead of the overall environment—and so hotels unwittingly or not end up marketing their mattresses.

Bed and bedding have become luxury items, incorporating a wide range of new materials and technology with escalating prices to match. Electronic sensors and heating and cooling systems are now being built into mattresses. If you can afford them, go ahead, splurge on yourself and your family. Hopefully you will sleep great. But if you are having trouble sleeping in the first place, is a new mattress the answer? If your old, lumpy mattress is clearly in need of replacing, sure, but otherwise, probably not.

Think back to how you slept as a child. You could blissfully fall asleep on the floor of a friend's home with just a blanket and pillow. As a teenager, you were happy sleeping on a friend's couch. There is very little independent scientific data that suggests that changing mattresses makes a difference in improving poor sleep for most people.

Stay Away from Used Mattresses

If at all possible, however, never buy a used mattress. After years of use, a mattress weighs *more* than it did when it was new. Let that sink in. The mattress gets heavier over time because it absorbs oil and sweat from skin. Dust mites can grow in the mattress by feeding on the dead skin that flakes off on the mattress. Dust mites can cause allergies. Allergies can cause . . . well, we're back to the sleep issue again.

Weighing In on Weighted Blankets

Weighted blankets have become increasingly popular, in particular for helping children with autistic spectrum disorder sleep better. The idea behind weighted blankets is that feeling more hugged or squeezed releases the hormone oxytocin, which is associated with social bonding and lowered anxiety. The popularity of weighted blankets has also spread as a remedy for other conditions, such as insomnia. I have met people who say their sleep is improved with weighted blankets, but no strong scientific evidence exists at this time showing that they make a difference in objective sleep measures. A randomized trial of children using weighted blankets did not find that they had increased or improved sleep, but the children did prefer them over normal blankets. If a weighted blanket helps you sleep better, by all means use one, but don't expect a magic-bullet fix for your insomnia.

Pillow Talk

When buying a pillow, look for one that conforms naturally to the contours of your head and neck, like a feather or memory-foam pillow. Pillows that are thick and firm may force your neck into an unnatural flexed position. So-called cervical pillows have built-in support to ergonomically align the neck and are contoured to cradle the natural curvature of shoulders, head, and neck. Japanese *sobakawa* pillows are filled with natural buckwheat hulls; they conform to the head and neck and maintain their firm shape. (Some people swear by sobakawa, while others liken it to sleeping on a crunchy bag of pebbles.)

People often claim they sleep only in a certain position, and pillow brands often market designs specifically to side sleepers, stomach sleepers, and back sleepers. But watch videos of people sleeping (which I do) and you'll observe that people change positions throughout the night. Trust me: Just because you end up in the same position you started sleeping in does not mean you were in that one position all night. In short, you might want to skip these designs.

An entire industry has grown up around body pillows for pregnancy. These are effective in helping a woman sleep on her side and shift some of the pressure off the back and hips and perhaps even help shift the weight off the aorta.

If you suffer from allergies to materials such as real feathers, hypoallergenic options—like those made of memory foam, bamboo, and polyester fiber—are your best bet.

Over-the-counter snoring remedies are many and varied, including "snore-alarm" pillows that gently vibrate when your snore reaches a certain decibel level, and smart pillows with tracking sensors that provide real-time sleep analysis. I've even seen pillows sold with motors inside that turn your head if a sensor detects snoring. By the time I see a patient for a sleep apnea evaluation, pillows are usually not enough (which is not to say there isn't a role for positional therapy for sleep apnea; see page 36).

As the sleep epidemic grows, it's no surprise that more gimmicky pillow options are hitting the market. In addition to the previously mentioned "snoring remedies," so-called magnetic pillows containing magnets are marketed as therapeutic for pain and other ills, but the medical claims are dubious. And because the magnets can interfere with the function of pacemaker devices, individuals with pacemakers should avoid magnetic pillows completely. "Cooling pillows," using cooling gel and memory-foam technology, appeal to those who "sleep hot" or suffer from night sweats. Each of these pillows may work for somebody, but they don't work for everyone.

Scent and Sleep

You may not think that something as ethereal and fleeting as scent would have much impact on our sleep, but evidence shows that aromatherapy can have some benefits. The smell of lavender, for example, is reported to have a calming effect and was shown to provide subjective improvements in sleep in multiple studies. This is because when we fall asleep, our brain goes through a process of perceptual disengagement as it turns inward, becoming less responsive to external stimuli. But one sense does remain "online" even when we are deeply asleep: our sense of smell, a holdover from prehistoric times when we needed to be alert to predators' scents.

Keep in mind that using aromatherapy—whether through a scented mist on your pillow or a room diffuser—can be a pleasant way to drift off to sleep, but it is likeliest to help only those with mild sleep problems.

Dogs May Help You Sleep Better

Dogs have been warning humans about predators for thousands of years, from prehistoric days when we were vulnerable to attack from big cats while we slept to modern times when backyard dogs

dogs sound the alarm if intruders are present. Dogs see more clearly in dimmer light and sense motion better than humans. They also have shorter sleep cycles and wake up more often than we do at night. It's no surprise, then, that people—and in particular, women—sleep better when dogs are in the bedroom. Add in the intense love and devotion dogs have for humans (and vice versa), and you can see why they can be ideal bedroom companions. Plus, having to let the dog out in the morning helps train humans to have a consistent wake-up time.

EVERYDAY SLEEP ISSUES

How to Sleep on a Plane

I have slept on many planes, usually in coach. Sleep is never guaranteed to us on any flight, no matter where we sit—although ever-shrinking economy-class seats can make even a nap a serious challenge. Before every flight, I think about whether I plan to sleep and, if so, what I need to do to prepare. Here are my recommendations:

- **Skip caffeine** altogether during the day if you plan to sleep on the flight.

- **Wear loose clothing and shoes you can easily slip off** (but always keep your socks on!).

- If lights keep you from sleeping, **bring along an eye mask.**

- If the noises inherent in flying (cockpit announcements, jet-engine sonics) bother you, **carry noise-canceling headphones or earplugs.** I prefer headphones—I find them more useful, more comfortable, and safer than earplugs, because periodically you need to hear what is happening around you, and the crew and fellow passengers can tell more easily that you are sound isolated. Headphones also give you the option of entertainment if you like falling asleep listening to music, say, or a podcast.

- Especially if you're traveling alone, **don't take sleeping pills on the flight.** Doing so leaves you less responsive to your surroundings and potentially vulnerable. If the effects of the sleeping pill last longer than the flight, then disembarking at your destination can also pose potential problems—especially if you plan to drive once you're off the plane.

- If you have a tendency to snore, **skip the in-flight cocktail.** Drinking alcohol can make your snoring louder, a sound that really echoes throughout the plane.

- If you use one, **bring your CPAP machine.** Modern CPAP devices are FAA-approved for in-flight use. You might feel self-conscious at first, but your fellow passengers probably won't mind if the alternative is loud snoring.

- Most airplane seats are not designed for sleeping, and falling asleep in unnatural positions can result in neck discomfort. To make matters worse, when we enter sleep, our neck muscles relax and the sudden drop in our head position when sleeping sitting up can jolt us awake. **A travel pillow will provide extra support** so you can sleep better sitting up, keeping your head and neck in alignment and reducing neck strain.

Jet Lag: Time-Shifting in a Modern World

Because the human circadian clock evolved to make gradual changes over the course of the year, it can't handle abrupt switches in time zones. This is why we experience jet lag: Our inner clock becomes out of sync with the world around us, resulting in a sleep schedule that is notably disrupted. Other body rhythms, such as eating schedules, are also disturbed, and we often feel unwell, suffering from symptoms like irritability, malaise, and headaches.

As a general rule, your circadian clock takes about one day of adjustment per time zone traveled. So a traveler zipping through three time zones should expect to feel out of sorts for about three days. (If you are planning a trip that is fewer than three days, you will feel better if you simply stay on the schedule of your home time zone.) Luckily, for longer trips, there are proven strategies for correcting jet lag and minimizing the ill effects of abrupt time shifts:

- **Expose yourself to as much light as possible** soon after waking up the first morning in your new destination.

- **Do some physical exercise** in the afternoon to push away the surge in drowsiness.

- **Stay hydrated and avoid alcohol.** Staying hydrated is a good practice in low-humidity environments like that aboard planes. Alcohol makes changing time zones even harder, especially if you are already sleep deprived (see page 60 for more on alcohol's effect on sleep).

- **If you're traveling east,** you are shortening your day and bedtime comes earlier than your biological clock is used to. Start adjusting to the expected new time zone by going to sleep early in the days before you begin the trip. Try not to nap during your flight so you'll have an easier time falling asleep in your new time zone. Avoid bright light as much as possible when you land—you want your brain to anticipate the earlier nighttime. If you're taking an overnight flight east and arriving at your destination in the early-morning hours, then you'll maximize your exposure to light in the new time zone, helping you stay awake.

- **If you're traveling west,** you are prolonging your day, so catching a brief nap on the flight can help you stay alert in your new time zone. It's usually easier to adapt to traveling west than traveling east because staying up later is easier than going to bed early.

- **If your trip is five days or fewer and you prefer to keep a schedule consistent with your home time zone:** Our circadian tendency toward sleepiness hits us about two hours before our usual wake-up time. When you are approaching this point in your new time zone, take a nap to help keep you on a sleep schedule similar to the one you have at home.

- **If jet lag is significantly hindering your ability to function,** the short-term use of hypnotics or stimulants either alone or in combination can be helpful to adapt to a new schedule. These can be taken, in consultation with your physician, for a few days while you're in your new destination and a few days upon returning home.

Spring Forward, Fall Back

Even a one-hour time change can take days to recover from, much like a mini jet lag. Daylight saving time is a prime example. We don't necessarily sleep a full hour more the evening we set our clocks back, and we certainly don't tend to spring to our feet the morning after we've set our clocks forward. In fact, it takes some of us up to five full days to get back to our baseline selves after daylight saving time goes into effect. You can help mitigate the of time change, such as fatigue and drowsiness, by gradually adjusting your sleep routine in the week or two before.

To prepare to "spring forward," start by going to bed fifteen minutes earlier than you usually do and getting out of bed fifteen minutes earlier. After a few days, if you are able to fall asleep easily and wake up on time, repeat the process. Do this in reverse in anticipation of "falling back." Adjusting your routine gradually is an easier, gentler way to extend total sleep time. And seek out natural light as much as possible when you first wake up. Sunlight helps reset your biological clock.

Sometimes It Makes Sense Not to Sleep

To the brain, stress and danger are similar, so it makes biological sense that the brain will avoid sleeping during stressful situations—whether a family member has suddenly taken ill, you suffer an unexpected loss of income, or your job is on the line. Even trying to sleep the first time your teenager spends a late night out can stress you out. When faced with the worst of life's myriad curveballs, it would be strange if you *could* sleep well. Short-term inability to sleep is a natural occurrence that can happen to any one of us. But if poor sleep continues for several weeks, speak with your health-care provider.

FIVE

SLEEP DISORDERS

SLEEP DISORDERS CAN happen at any age. The good news is that the majority improve with the right approach. Obstructive sleep apnea and insomnia are the disorders we see most in sleep-medicine clinics, and those are discussed in detail in chapters two and three, respectively. There are more than eighty recognized clinical sleep disorders, however, so in the pages that follow I'll offer a brief overview of other common ones.

Narcolepsy

We spend our entire lives awake, dreaming, or sleeping but not dreaming. In sleep medicine, we describe these states of the brain as wake, REM sleep, and NREM sleep (for more, see page 14). When the switching mechanism between these three states becomes unstable, elements of sleep can intrude into the awake state, and vice versa. This is what happens when a person develops narcolepsy, a neurological disorder that usually begins in childhood or young adulthood. People with narcolepsy can be irresistibly sleepy, able to fall asleep most anywhere, even during a meal or in the middle of conversation. They may have bouts of sleep paralysis (see page 91). One remarkable aspect of narcolepsy is that elements of dreaming can intrude into the awake state. When this happens, a person may have hallucinations so vivid that they call 911.

The most unique feature of narcolepsy is a phenomenon called cataplexy. Normally when we dream, a signal in our brain switches off the movement of most of our muscles. With cataplexy, something similar happens. When a narcoleptic person is suddenly excited or laughs, some of their muscles briefly lose tone. It can be as subtle as a mild facial droop or as extreme as a fall to the ground. Although they may appear to have fainted, they are actually conscious and aware of what is happening around them.

Because the initial manifestations of narcolepsy can be subtle, especially in children, it can take years—and extensive unnecessary tests or treatments—to zero in on the right diagnosis. The phenomenon is hard to describe and even harder to believe. The hallucinations are often mischaracterized as psychosis and the sleepiness as attention deficit disorder. One of my youngest patients with narcolepsy told me that the first time she noticed something was wrong was when she was eight years old and playing soccer. When the ball came to her, she was excited to see an open net. But instead of kicking the ball, she fell down. People laughed and thought she had slipped, but as she told her mother, "I didn't slip." The girl went on to undergo an extensive medical workup, including testing for Lyme disease and seizures, no doubt a frightening and expensive ordeal for both her and her family. But if doctors had listened to what she was saying from the very beginning, they would have realized she was perfectly describing cataplexy.

Narcolepsy is often misdiagnosed as a psychiatric or emotional problem, but it's a real neurological condition. Fortunately, once diagnosed, effective treatment is available, starting with simply taking a short nap every day.

Sleeping with Your Eyes Open

Sleeping with your eyes open or partially open occurs in an estimated 10 to 20 percent of the population. For sleep partners, it can be a disconcerting sight. Nocturnal lagophthalmos, the inability to close the eyelids while sleeping, is generally harmless but can cause dry, irritated eyes and may lead to more serious problems, such as eye infections and impaired vision. If you find you're always waking up with red, dry, or irritated eyes, see your doctor, who can prescribe a topical treatment, among other remedies. If you suddenly start sleeping with your eyes open, it may be a symptom of a thyroid, dermatological, or neurological condition, and you should seek medical evaluation.

Sleepwalking

The brain is such a complex structure that it shouldn't be surprising that one part of the brain can be in one state while another area is in another state. That's when things really get weird—we can sleepwalk and do all kinds of things without being fully awake. Sleepwalkers may eat things they would not normally eat or engage in sex differently than while they're awake. People have also been reported to rearrange furniture in their sleep, among other seemingly complex behaviors. Some might even turn on their cars and try to drive!

An arousal disorder, sleepwalking tends to occur during our deepest NREM sleep, when the most rational part of our brain (the prefrontal cortex) is less active but we can still carry out behaviors we've done over and over, such as walking or trying to cook or drive a car. Couldn't you put the key in the ignition, turn on the car, and shift it into gear with your eyes closed? (You won't drive well, however.) Sleepwalking episodes may occur more often in certain stressful situations, such as when traveling or sleeping in a different place, or when a child is ill with a fever.

There is a strong genetic component to sleepwalking, and sleepwalkers often have a family history of other arousal disorders, like sleep terrors (see page 93). Sleepwalking is most common in children ages six to eight and typically disappears after adolescence. Treatment of young sleepwalkers is usually unnecessary, although you'll want to take precautionary measures to minimize the potential for injury (such as putting up gates to stairs or removing sharp objects) if your child is a habitual sleepwalker.

Adult cases are much less common, occurring in about 1 to 2 percent of the population, but can be more difficult to treat. In general, any person with violent, atypical, or treatment-resistant sleepwalking should be seen by a sleep-medicine specialist. Intriguingly, hypnosis can be an effective treatment for some sleepwalkers.

Common wisdom (and many a sitcom plotline) says that it's dangerous to wake a sleepwalker. It is not dangerous *for the sleepwalker* to be woken, but it is dangerous (and difficult) for you to wake them! In the grip of a deep sleep, sleepwalkers are not in a rational state of mind and can injure you if you get in their way. Sleepwalkers don't feel pain the same way as when they are awake. For adult sleepwalkers, take safety precautions—such as hanging draperies to keep the sleepwalker from cutting themselves on broken glass if they break a window, installing an alarm system that can notify others if the sleepwalker leaves the home, and removing weapons that are within easy access of the sleepwalker. In fact, simply having the person sleep in a light sleeping bag on top of the bed may restrict the person's movements sufficiently to keep him or her safe. Never tie down or lock a sleepwalker in a room, in case of an emergency such as a fire or an earthquake.

Sleep Paralysis

The first time I experienced sleep paralysis, I was studying in the medical school library and fell asleep with my arms draped across my books. I was obviously sleep deprived, because I hadn't been out for long when I began to have an intense dream. As I started to drift into a nightmare, I jerked awake but found I was unable to lift my head or arms!

It turns out, being sleep deprived makes us do strange things. During normal dreaming/REM sleep, we cannot move most of our muscles from the neck down. It's not that those muscles are merely relaxed. Rather, an active signal is traveling down our spinal cord to stop those muscles from moving. Even some of our reflexes shut down. Sometimes these processes are not perfectly coordinated, and when we transition abruptly from dreaming to being awake, we gain consciousness before the signal to stop our muscle movements has completely lifted. Sleep paralysis is often felt in the chest area and in some cultures is described as a ghost sitting on one's chest! It can be a scary phenomenon but it's usually fleeting.

Falling Asleep and Jerking Yourself Awake

In the transition from wake to sleep, many odd things can happen. In addition to sleep paralysis, another is the sensation of falling and suddenly jerking yourself awake. If you are in bed (sending the message to your body that you want to sleep) but at the same time resisting sleep by thinking or reading, you are giving your body mixed signals. This mixed message can cause our bodies to misfire and experience these odd sensations, collectively called hypnic jerks, or sleep starts. If you are in bed and having these sensations, stop whatever you are doing and just go to sleep. Your body is telling you what it needs.

Talking in Your Sleep

A normal variant of human sleep, sleep talking (called somniloquy) is not dangerous. Sleep talking can happen at any time in the night and is not necessarily linked to dreams. If you have a tendency to talk in your sleep, let your sleep partner or whoever hears you know that whatever you say is generally nonsensical—in other words, what you say may or may not be true. You are not revealing some deep, dark secrets while you sleep. (Well, *maybe* you're not. Early on in my relationship with my wife, she told me she knew I loved her because after an argument she heard me say so in my sleep. I did not argue the point and was glad I made her happy.)

Abrupt yelling during sleep, usually combined with restless or even violent behavior, warrants further investigation, however. It could be a harmless sleep terror episode (see below), but it could also be something more serious, such as a seizure or neurodegenerative disorder. So if you have never had any vocal outbursts in your sleep and abruptly start to do so as you get older, let your physician know.

Sleep Terrors

A sleep terror is an abnormal event characterized by a sleeping person suddenly sitting up and letting out a bloodcurdling scream. Their eyes may be wide open, but staring straight past you. The person will be agitated and inconsolable but after a few minutes will lie back down and resume sleeping peacefully like nothing unusual happened. The next morning the person will have no memory of the previous night's event, but anyone who witnessed it won't be able to forget it.

Unlike nightmares, which are more likely to occur during REM sleep and to be vividly remembered by the dreamer the next day, sleep terrors tend to occur in the first third of the night, waking one out of their deepest slow-wave (N3) sleep. What happens is that during this deep stage of sleep, the part of the brain that deals with rational thought (the prefrontal cortex) is hard to rouse. But another part of the brain, the limbic system, can become activated. This part of the brain is involved in our fight-or-flight reactions; since the rational part of our brain is offline, it cannot control the limbic system, which is then free to direct the body to behave wildly, or even violently.

Sleep terrors are more common in children, but some adults have them, too. For the most part, children outgrow sleep terrors. Children with sleep terrors may also sleepwalk (see page 90), so if sleepwalking runs in the family, be mindful that a child experiencing sleep terrors may get out of bed at some point.

Night Gnashing

Many of us unintentionally gnash or grind our teeth while we sleep—a medical condition known as sleep bruxism. It can make an awful sound (and can be very disturbing to a bed partner), but worse, it may lead to pain in the temporomandibular joint (TMJ) and do damage to your teeth.

Bruxism, which can occur during the day or at night, is frequently associated with a preexisting dental or jaw problem. When one's upper and lower teeth are not properly aligned, they don't don't interlock during sleep. The grinding sound of bruxism is caused by the teeth gliding past one another. Tooth grinding is often associated with stress and is particularly common in children, but it may also occur as a side effect of commonly used psychiatric medications and some antidepressants. Alcohol can exacerbate the problem, as it prevents us from entering REM, the sleep of dreams; studies show that we don't usually grind our teeth when we dream. Untreated obstructive sleep apnea may also aggravate any tendencies toward bruxism.

If you're waking up with jaw pain or headaches, bruxism may be a cause. Contact your dentist for a comprehensive dental examination. To prevent further dental and jaw damage, you may be outfitted with a mouthguard to wear over your teeth while you sleep. The use of Botox injections around the jawline has also provided temporary relief for some people. If your bed partner tells you that you are grinding your teeth at night, don't ignore it. Treating bruxism can not only prevent a lot of pain, but it can also save your relationship!

Restless Leg Syndrome

Restless leg syndrome (RLS) is a movement disorder first described more than four hundred years ago. Back then, people with RLS symptoms feared a curse had been put upon them. Even today, patients with RLS often say it feels like a curse—the disorder seems designed to drive someone insane. Those afflicted feel an urge to move when they are resting. The feeling goes away as long as they are moving and working, but recurs when they try to rest, especially in bed at night.

One of the most common sleep disorders, RLS can start at any age. The severity of the symptoms fluctuates a great deal from patient to patient but tends to be more severe in middle or old age. Some patients may go years without feeling any RLS symptoms, and many women first become aware of the disorder when symptoms flare up during pregnancy.

Restless leg syndrome can be tricky to diagnose. The legs appear normal, there are no other physical signs that something is amiss, and no laboratory tests can pin down the diagnosis. One clue that you may be suffering from RLS: You have a family history of the disorder. The prevalence of RLS among first-degree relatives of RLS sufferers is three to five times greater than that of the general population. It is uncommon to find a patient with RLS who does not have another family member afflicted by it. These family members might not even know they have the condition or simply think it is normal because many of their relatives have it.

RLS can improve with treatment, such as behavioral or lifestyles changes like limiting nighttime caffeine, running a cold cloth along the legs before bed, taking a warm bath, doing some stretching exercises before bed, or going for an evening walk. (I sometimes wonder how many of my late-night dog-walking neighbors have RLS.) Simply moving the legs may temporarily improve the sensation. Note that moderate exercise at night can make it better, but strenuous exercise can actually make it worse. Medications (such as dopamine agonists) and iron supplements can also be very effective in treating RLS.

Delayed Sleep Phase Syndrome

Delayed sleep phase syndrome (DSPS) is one of the most common sleep disorders among adolescents, perhaps second only to that age group's classic issues with insufficient sleep. DSPS is characterized by difficulty falling asleep without difficulty staying asleep. It's a circadian disorder, meaning the problem is in the *timing* of sleep. Young people with DSPS sleep fine when they can set their own schedules. Where they run into trouble is when they have to sleep on a schedule imposed on them. People with DSPS often think of themselves as night owls, but most of us who sleep later than usual on weekends can return to our usual weekday schedule without much difficulty. People with DSPS have a harder time making this adjustment.

DSPS starts to show in adolescence and young adulthood because this is when we have more personal freedom, without enforced bedtimes and with the ability to sleep in dramatically on weekends. The syndrome can persist into adulthood if a person's lifestyle or occupation allows them to be up at night or have very flexible hours. For many others, having a more structured work environment or raising kids of their own will force them to synchronize their sleep schedule to a more conventional time. But when they have extended time off, they may revert to a DSPS sleeping pattern.

DSPS was first described in 1981 in a group of young adults who were thought to have an atypical form of depression. They seemed to be depressed, but they did not respond to antidepressants and had a different sleep pattern than is usually seen in typical depression. With depression, people generally wake up too early and can't get back to sleep, whereas the DSPS patients slept just fine once they fell asleep. But because they fell asleep *later* than expected, they had a hard time getting up in the morning. These young people with DSPS got dramatically better when their sleep schedules were realigned to fit their school or work schedules.

Bright-light exposure in the morning (phototherapy) and locking in a wake-up schedule on weekends that is as close to their weekday schedule as possible for several weeks can help shift a person with DSPS back into a more traditional sleep schedule. It is important to consult your doctor about the possibility of an undiagnosed sleep disorder in any young person who appears to have depression, especially if sleep is atypical.

SIX

A LIFETIME OF SLEEPING WELL

WE ALL KNOW the importance of eating well and maintaining our physical fitness, but getting a solid night's sleep is as vital to a lifetime of good health as any of those. This chapter looks at sleep throughout the stages of life, from newborns to adolescents to the elderly, and addresses how we can sleep better at every age.

As you'll see in the following pages, poor sleep has no age, social, or cultural boundaries. It's never too early or too late to acquire better habits. I have had the privilege of helping people in all different stages of life learn to sleep well and wake up refreshed.

Infant Sleep

Few things create more apprehension for expectant parents than getting their babies to sleep. Those who already have children almost gleefully bring up the terrors of sleep deprivation to new parents, and one of the first things a stranger asks the mother or father of a newborn is "How does your baby sleep?"

Of course, many parents hear that question as "How good a parent are you turning out to be?" Some smugly announce their child is *already* sleeping through the night, while others bemoan their "bad sleeper." The truth is, just like adults (see page 18), *no* babies sleep through the night—some are just waking up their parents more often than others. If a baby that sleeps seven hours a night is born to a parent used to sleeping eight hours a night (before they had a child), they will complain bitterly that their baby is a bad sleeper. Take that same seven-hour sleeping baby born to a parent who sleeps six hours, and they will brag about how their child sleeps through the night! They will freely give advice to other parents and become the kings and queens of the local new parents' group. Yet in both cases the child is sleeping the same number of hours.

From the moment you learn you will be a parent, you have something to worry about. That never seems to go away. When I meet new parents in my office, I sometimes ask them how old they were when their own parents stopped worrying about them. The answer, of course, is pretty much never. Learning to live with these uncertainties and worries is a challenge for all parents. My strongest piece of advice is to think of your child not as a "good" sleeper or a "bad" sleeper. However your child might sleep, it is a learned behavior, and together you'll tailor an approach and a schedule that works best for you and your child.

A SLEEP DOCTOR'S FIRST CHILD

I became established early in my career at Stanford as an expert in children's sleep, based on my specialized medical training in child neurology and a formal fellowship in sleep medicine. Then I had my daughter. The holy grail of parenting an infant is getting your new baby to "sleep through the night." I was considered an expert, but I had a lot to learn.

The best-known physician on children's sleep was (and is) Dr. Richard Ferber. His famed Ferberization, or Ferber method, calls for letting babies "cry it out" when they wake intermittently during the night (as all infants do), without their parents' intervention. It is based on the concept that there is a learned component to sleeping, and that babies learn to associate certain activities with sleeping. For example, if a child is rocked to sleep in their parent's arms, then when the baby awakens at night, they need to be rocked again, since that's how they learned to fall asleep in the first place. So Dr. Ferber argued that if parents want their baby to learn to fall back to sleep without their help, they should put the baby down in the crib *before* they actually fall asleep and not scoop them up every time they cry out. This way, so the theory goes, the baby learns to fall asleep on their own.

It all made sense—that is, until my daughter was born. As a sleep physician, I was eager to test the validity of Dr. Ferber's process. So I broke his rules on purpose. I rocked my daughter to sleep, then put her in her crib. She slept fine. I let her fall asleep in her crib, then picked her up and brought her into our bed. She still slept fine. I let her fall asleep in our bed, then moved her to her crib. She continued to sleep fine. She would be sleeping, I would poke her awake, she would look at me and go back to sleep. Despite my annoyances, she slept soundly and was sleeping through the night by the time she was eight weeks old without requiring nighttime nursing or interventions.

About a year later, I was invited to participate in a panel with Dr. Ferber himself. Before the panel began, I sheepishly introduced myself. Almost apologetically, I told him I had broken his rules with my daughter and she still slept well. He calmly smiled and said, "That happens sometimes." It was not what I was expecting him to say. It was only much later, with the birth of my son, that I realized how insightful his comment was.

INFANT SLEEP: CASE STUDY 2

A SLEEP DOCTOR'S SECOND CHILD

When our son was born, my confidence as a sleep expert had grown into a swagger. No need to experiment; I knew what I was doing. My wife had also been studying sleep and would become a sleep-medicine physician herself. But our new baby son quickly brought us both back to reality.

In the first few weeks of our son's life, he cried inconsolably, often at night. None of us was sleeping well. What to do? I wasn't sure I wanted my coworkers at the sleep clinic to know what we were going through—I was the sleep expert, after all. I certainly couldn't call Dr. Ferber after telling him I ignored his rules and everything turned out fine!

One night, just as my wife and I had fallen asleep, our son's crying pierced the quiet. Determined to fix the problem once and for all, I went to his room and held him. He kept crying. In my sleep-deprived state, I started thinking about inventing something to help my son sleep better, something womblike, perhaps a system with a large bag where he could be immersed upside down in warm fluid and provided oxygen at the same time. (In my semidelirious mind this was making sense to me.) Then I remembered that I had a new CD, Bob Dylan's *Time Out of Mind*, that I might as well listen to since I was up with the baby anyway. Within moments of putting on the CD, my son stopped crying. *I must contact Bob Dylan about making a children's album*, I thought to myself in my sleep-deprived state. *There must be something about the frequency of the sound of his voice that calms children.* I went so far as to wonder if Bob Dylan would actually participate in research to see why his voice helps babies sleep.

Then it hit me: The CD had calmed *me* down. The music was making me sway rhythmically, and that in turn calmed my baby boy. After that night, my son started sleeping better, and he was sleeping through the night by six weeks, even faster than his sister.

Any experienced parent will tell you that each child is different. But with each child the parent is also different. "It happens sometimes"—Dr. Ferber's words to a new father, me, were insightful indeed.

Co-sleeping: Not for Infants, but Okay for Toddlers!

The American Academy of Pediatrics (AAP) has strongly recommended that during the first year of life a baby should not sleep in the same bed as their parents because of the increased risk of sudden unexpected infant death (SUID), one of the leading causes of mortality in infants. The AAP recommends that babies sleep in a separate, firm space on their backs. Bedding—including blankets, pillows, or stuffed toys—should be kept out of their sleeping area. The AAP further recommends that infants sleep in the same *room* with their parents, to help promote nursing and ensure overall safety.

The distinction between co-sleeping and sleeping separately is not as black and white as it's made out to be, though. Snuggling with our young children is one of the most unique aspects of parenting, and an experience we cherish and often miss when they grow older. Family photos of parents sleeping with their children portray an irresistible, intimate sweetness. Allowing toddlers or older children to get into bed with you in the middle of the night (after a bad dream, or when they're feeling unwell), or to share a bed with you when grandparents come to visit or when staying at a hotel, is a perfectly fine and safe practice.

Traveling with Babies and Small Children

Imagine you are sitting in your economy seat waiting for the plane to fill up, when a young mother appears in the regular boarding line, traveling alone with a young infant and carting a stroller and carry-on luggage. She is already stressed from missing preboarding, and she knows she will have to hold the baby in her arms the entire flight. She is hoping that her seatmate will be someone who likes kids and is not going to get her baby sick. As they watch the mother moving slowly down the aisle, everyone next to an empty seat avoids making eye contact with the mother. *If I look away,* they think, *the seat next to mine will stay empty.* The tension in the cabin builds. Suddenly the infant starts to cry, and it echoes throughout the plane. Now all eyes are on the mother.

Nobody wants to be *that parent,* dealing with a crying baby on a plane. But it happens. My wife and I traveled often with our children when they were very young because we regularly attended the same medical conferences, so I know from firsthand experience that you can't always control the situation—you can only try to prevent or mitigate any meltdowns. I've found that you travel better with young children when you consider the following:

- **Take full advantage of any preboarding opportunities.** It provides extra time to unload carry-on luggage into overhead bins and get your kids settled in.

- Depending on your destination and length of the trip, **plan the timing of sleep in advanc**e. We all know that children get cranky if they stay awake past their usual bedtime or naptime. If your children are old enough to understand, let them know beforehand that they will be sleeping on the plane. Have them board wearing their pajamas, and don't forget any transitional objects they like to sleep with. Ear muffs or noise-canceling headphones, which are available in small sizes, can also help them get to sleep (earplugs are not recommended for young children, as they can be a choking hazard).

- **Always discuss the possibility of using medication with your pediatrician first.** In general, you'll want to avoid prescription sleep aids unless your doctor recommends them. If you do decide to give your child sleeping medication, whether a prescription or an over-the-counter remedy, be sure to test it a few days before the trip, at the same time you'd give your child the medication on the day of travel. Sometimes medication meant to help a child sleep can cause a paradoxical reaction if given at an unusual time of the day. This can happen especially with over-the-counter antihistamines. It can also occur with prescription sleep aids.

- **Prepare your kids for "airplane ear."** Tell older children that when the plane is taking off or landing, their ears may hurt, but chewing on something yummy (or drinking something) will help them feel better, and it all goes away fast. Consider nursing or giving an infant a bottle at both takeoff and landing (anything that makes the baby move their jaw will help them equalize the pressure in their ears).

- If you prefer that your children stay awake on the plane (so they can sleep on schedule at their destination), **have a plan to entertain them.** Let them watch movies or draw. Bring along favorite snacks and books. If more than one child is traveling together, have them sit side-by-side so they can interact. You may be surprised how well they play together when they have no other choice.

- Above all else, **don't get upset**. There is a possibility they may not sleep at all, given the novelty and excitement of the airplane. If you project calm, your children will pick up on it and stay calm, too.

TRAVELING WITH CHILDREN: CASE STUDY

A CRYING BABY ON A PLANE

A neighbor of mine once took a flight to Oklahoma to visit her parents so they could meet their new grandchild. She was traveling alone with her infant daughter and the baby was crying through the entire boarding process and continued to wail as they took off. After the plane leveled, the pilot came out of the cockpit and said, "Where is that baby?" She came over to the mother and asked to hold her daughter. In her arms, the girl calmed down immediately and stopped crying. The rest of the passengers on the plane started to applaud. My neighbor was relieved and embarrassed at the same time. The pilot, naturally, had to return to the cockpit. When she handed the baby back to the mom, her daughter started crying again. My neighbor told me it felt like the longest flight of her life.

But of course the pilot didn't have a magic touch. She was simply more relaxed and used to the routine of flying with cranky passengers (of all ages!). The baby was sensing the mother's stress and reacting to it by crying.

All of us sleep best in a state of serenity. If your baby is otherwise healthy but is crying, regardless of how public or tense the situation, the best thing you can do is to take a deep breath.

Note—this advice applies to older children, too! No matter how frustrated you feel, yelling is rarely going to succeed in helping them get a good night's sleep.

How Many Hours Should My Child Sleep?

Whenever I speak to a group of parents, someone inevitably asks how many hours their child should sleep. Since the time during which a child is asleep is the closest parents usually get to the freedom they had before they had children, I wonder if what they are really asking is how much of a reprieve will they get from the hectic life of parenting! Here are some general guidelines:

- The range reported for infants is wide, and when you factor in naps can be from **eleven to eighteen hours** of total daily sleep.

- By age three, toddlers are starting to give up naps, and their total sleep time ranges from **ten to sixteen hours.**

- In general, **nine to ten hours** is a healthy amount of sleep for most school-age children.

- As children age they gradually need less sleep, but with the onset of puberty individual adolescents may need more sleep than they did when they were younger, from **eight and a half to nine and a half hours.** The majority of teenagers are sleeping less than the recommended amount.

There is one important caveat to all of this, though: As discussed on page 20, some people inherently require less sleep than others. If an infant or child has the genetic tendencies of a shorter-sleeping parent but is spending the bulk of their time with a longer-sleeping parent, that parent may complain about how little the child sleeps. The child may grow up being told they are a bad sleeper. Or a parent may put their child to bed too early, making them feel frustrated for being forced into bed when they're not sleepy. This can set up a lifetime of sleeping problems, and the child's self-esteem may suffer from their inability to sleep in such a way as to please their mom or dad. So if your child seems to have difficulty meeting the general guidelines for the number of hours sleeping but appears to be alert, well rested, and energetic throughout the day without requiring naps, the problem may be you, not them!

Get the Jump on Toddler Sleep Problems

Most toddlers sleep great. They wake up refreshed and happy and have amazing energy all day long. The toddler years are also the time when sleep disorders can emerge, however. Some disorders, like sleepwalking (see page 90) and sleep terrors (see page 93), tend to improve as a child gets older. Conditions such as obstructive sleep apnea (see page 31), however, may gradually worsen over time.

Snoring, restless sleep, or mouth breathing can indicate potential problems—especially if either parent has a sleep disorder—and you should not wait for your toddler to outgrow these conditions. Snoring among preschoolers is a great predictor of being labeled as having attention deficit disorder (ADD) upon entry to elementary school. "Growing pains" in toddlers, often a symptom of restless leg syndrome (see page 95), can also result in an ADD misdiagnosis. Nighttime fears and bedtime refusal may later transform into a pattern of chronic insomnia. Take heart: All of these conditions can be improved upon with proper attention, so get the jump on problematic sleep disorders early by speaking first to your pediatrician and then, if necessary, a sleep clinician.

TODDLER SLEEP: CASE STUDY

SLEEPING MAKES ME TIRED

My three-year-old patient looked me in the eye and said, "Doctor, sleeping makes me tired." His mother was perplexed. She told me that her son slept more than his friends, some of whom had already stopped napping. But he was always tired. Upon examining the boy, I saw right away that his tonsils were huge and no doubt blocked his breathing as he slept. The more he slept, the less he was breathing! So sleeping really did make him tired. He had his tonsils removed and got better quickly.

If your child is tired regardless of the number of hours they sleep, the problem is with their quality of sleep. Contact your child's physician to set up an overnight sleep study, which measures the quality of your child's sleep, for answers. (See page 144 for more on sleep studies.)

Fear and Sleep

Sleeping is a paradox, in which our bodies require us to both relax *and* do something that potentially puts us in a vulnerable situation, so it is easy to understand that for any of us, sleep and fear can naturally intersect. This is especially true for children. Teaching them that they are safe at night, in the dark, is essential to helping them sleep better, free of fearful thoughts. One piece of advice I give parents when they ask about bedtime fears is to avoid validating an irrational fear. If your child is scared of monsters, talk about monsters. In the popular children's book *Where the Wild Things Are* by Maurice Sendak, the central character, Max, is sent to his room as punishment. He has an imaginary dream adventure where he travels to an island full of monsters. But the monsters are scared of *him,* and later they learn to play together. I like how the book teaches that scary thoughts can be changed and we can learn to master our feelings.

On the other hand, if your child tells you there is a monster in the closet, don't go looking for one. You will only reinforce the possibility that there really is a monster there, and even worse, the monster has outsmarted you, the parent, by evading you! A similar approach can be applied to night-lights. It's one thing if a night-light is actually needed to see at night, but quite another if a child demands a light because of fear of the dark. In the latter case, teach them that it's safe to be in the dark inside their rooms. You can tell them that children throughout history (perhaps focusing on an era they happen to like) did not have night-lights. You can confide that you used to be scared of the dark, too, but now prefer it for sleeping. You can point out that leaving the lights on wastes electricity and is bad for the environment. You can show them that in fact we *can* still see without a light, once our eyes adjust to the darkness. Try to keep from making compromises, such as leaving a light on in the hallway. The point is for your child to learn that they are safe and to trust that their loving parent will keep them that way, day and night.

I am not saying you should ignore children's fears and make them tough it out. On the contrary, we need to listen to our children and help them understand that they can learn to sleep in the dark just like their parents and older siblings do. Note that if a child's nighttime anxiety is strong and resistant to changes, professional help may be needed. Childhood anxiety disorders are real conditions and should be treated by child psychologists and psychiatrists.

One other important thing: Never use your child's bedroom for time-outs or punishments. Sending children to bed early when they misbehave and letting them stay up late when they are good sends the wrong message. A child's sleep environment must be a sanctuary.

FEAR OF THE DARK

When my son was about four years old, he came home from preschool and announced that he was scared of the dark. I was surprised by this, since I had purposely played with him with flashlights in dark places, inside closets and under the bed, many times before and he never mentioned being fearful. So right away we went up to his room together. I closed the blinds and the door. We sat together in a rocking chair and I tossed a soft blanket over us. As we sat together, with him on my lap, I asked him how dark it was. "It's very dark," he said. "I can't see my hand." I asked him if he was afraid and he said no. I asked him why not and he sweetly said, "Because you are with me." Then I asked him if he was really afraid of the dark, or if perhaps he was afraid to be alone. "To be alone," he answered. I reassured him, telling him that "Even if you can't see us, you are never alone." We learn a lot from our children.

Nobody put their small children in separate caves or huts thirty thousand years ago. Sleeping separate from one's parents is a learned skill, just like wearing shoes or using a spoon. Most children are never in the dark alone except when they are in bed. Children thus learn to associate the dark with being alone. As parents, we need to teach them that they are safe and loved even if they cannot see us while they are sleeping. Let older toddlers understand that they can always trust you to keep them safe. Point out to them, for example, that when you take them on shopping trips, they go with you inside the store because it's safer than to leave them alone outside. Then explain that you let them sleep alone in a room because you know it is safe—in fact, their bedroom is the safest part of the home, as the front door of the house does not open into a bedroom. Hopefully, these reminders will help put any nascent fear of the dark to rest.

FEAR AND SLEEP: CASE STUDY 2

FORCE FIELD

A wealthy family came to our sleep clinic because their eight-year-old son was scared to go to sleep at night. "I don't know what's wrong," the father said, "Every night we walk around the house to show him the force field is turned on" (the "force field" being the household security system). "Why is the eight-year-old in charge of household security?" I asked.

There is a difference between *being* safe and *feeling* safe. I asked the boy if he had any doubts his parents loved him. "Of course not," he said. I asked him if his parents let him do things that are not safe, and he again laughingly said they didn't. When his parents write checks, I asked, does he question whether they have enough money in the bank? "No!" he responded to what he saw as yet another ridiculously obvious question. I pointed out that his answers showed that he was rightfully trusting of his parents and that he could count on them to keep him safe at night. To reinforce that, I asked his parents to continue to remind him that his bedroom is safe and that he doesn't need to do anything himself to make it so. His sleep improved, and he did not have to check the "force field" anymore.

Bed-Wetting

There are lots of reasons a child may need to urinate at night or have a bed-wetting accident. In determining the cause for bed-wetting, if your child is five years or older, you should first talk with your pediatrician to rule out any possible physical factors.

If your child is able to control their urination while awake but has always had persistent bed-wetting, it is likely a developmental issue, and possibly genetic. If the child previously woke up dry, for at least three months straight, but has now lost control, physical factors must be evaluated. Obstructive sleep apnea (see page 31) is an often-overlooked culprit when patients are told (erroneously) that stress is to blame. There are other rare possibilities that a physician may need to explore.

If a child is experiencing unusual stresses, psychological factors may be an issue, but most often that's not the case. I find it helpful to let the child know that they are not the only one in school with this problem, and that it even happens to much older children, including teenagers.

THE SLEEP APNEA–BED-WETTING CONNECTION

Many years ago I received a call about a teenage girl who had been admitted to the intensive-care unit after suffering a seizure, a bad reaction to a nasal spray that she had been prescribed to stop her chronic bed-wetting. I was called in by nurses in the ICU not for her bed-wetting issues but because the girl was snoring so loudly. It was clear from her symptoms and a follow-up sleep study that she was suffering from sleep apnea. She started receiving treatment for her sleep apnea and completely stopped bed-wetting a couple of days later!

Obstructive sleep apnea first emerges in children in the three- to six-year-old range, and based on the fact that this teen had been both snoring and unable to control her bed-wetting since age four, it's likely she had been suffering from untreated sleep apnea her entire childhood. The normal production of urine lessens when we sleep, meaning we can go longer without needing to urinate than when we are awake. But obstructive sleep apnea can cause a cascading series of events culminating in our kidneys making more urine at night, not less. If the signal to empty your bladder is strong enough, you will wake up to urinate. If you sleep through the signal, you wet the bed.

The teen was discharged from the hospital, and about ten years later I got a card from her, thanking me. She said that starting the treatment for sleep apnea had turned her life around. She had grown up blaming herself for bed-wetting as a child and being unable to go to slumber parties and sleepovers with her friends. Once her sleep apnea was diagnosed and treated, she realized the bed-wetting was not her fault. But I think she helped me more than I ever helped her. Hers was one of the first cases I saw that showed how sleep apnea as a cause of bed-wetting can be overlooked, even to this day.

Restless Leg Syndrome and Growing Pains

It should not hurt to grow. It has never been demonstrated that what have been coined as "growing pains," a generalized discomfort in the legs occurring most often in the evening, have anything to do with growth spurts. Instead, growing pains in a child may be a manifestation of a common neurological disorder known as restless leg syndrome (RLS)—see page 95. RLS strongly runs in families. If a child and a parent complain that their legs bother them at night, both likely suffer from RLS. The leg discomfort is often hard to describe, which is why it's sometimes characterized in children as "growing pains."

Restless leg syndrome can be very disruptive to a child's sleep and can result in daytime problems focusing, which can in turn lead to a misdiagnosis of attention deficit disorder. If your child complains of leg discomfort, particularly at night, and you have a family history of RLS, ask your physician for a sleep consult.

The Sleep-Deprived Adolescent

If you have a teenager in your life, you are probably dealing with a sleep-deprived person. The scientific data show that the majority of teenagers in the United States and many other countries are chronically sleep deprived. An average adolescent should sleep eight and a half to nine and a half hours per night to feel fully alert—but often sleeps far less. Teens frequently sleep for seven or fewer hours on school nights, according to the Centers for Disease Control and Prevention. This is why they sleep in so late on weekends, as their bodies try desperately to catch up on lost sleep. (Younger children usually get all the sleep they need during the school week and thus do not need to sleep in on weekends.)

We do something very unfair to teenagers. Even though they are still growing, we force them into a school system that does not allow them to get a full night of sleep. If you have a growing teenager or two, you know they can easily eat more than you. So it shouldn't be surprising that they need more sleep than you, too. Imagine if we controlled teenagers' access to food the same way we controlled their sleep schedules. We would partially starve them Monday through Friday, then tell them to eat as much as possible on the weekend, because come Monday we will be starving them again.

Adolescents as a group tend to stay up later and sleep later. Biology plays a big part in this: The onset of puberty causes a biological shift toward a tendency to a later sleep time. Research shows this occurs in other mammals as they mature, so it is not fair merely to pin it on your teen's cellphone or other screens. Young people often tell me they simply can't take a morning class because they are night owls. Behavioral factors, including homework loads, do play a role in adolescent night-owl behavior, however. Peer pressure can have a powerful influence, too: Teenagers don't usually brag to friends about how early they hit the sack every night. Staying awake past their parents' bedtime also satisfies teens' longing for privacy and autonomy.

Late-night-sleeping, exhausted adolescents can disrupt the entire household. Even worse, sleep deficit is known to have a profound negative impact on an adolescent's mental health, ability to drive safely, and academic and athletic performance. It's been proven to be an independent risk factor for car accidents and suicidal behavior, among the most common causes of death in this age group. This is why the American Academy of Pediatrics, among several other health organizations, has called for teenagers to start school no earlier than 8:30 a.m.

It is essential to teach your teens the importance of sleep, so they are motivated to make it a part of a healthy lifestyle. If they understand how important it is to their well-being, they are less likely to treat sleep as an inconvenience.

ADOLESCENT SLEEP: CASE STUDY

YOUNG-ADULT DROWSINESS IS A RED ALERT

The number-one cause of death for young adults is automobile accidents. For decades Stanford University students enrolled in Dr. Dement's Sleep and Dreams class have learned about this danger through a time-honored tradition: If a student falls asleep in class, they are squirted with water and upon awaking asked to shout the class motto "Drowsiness is red alert!"—after which they receive a round of applause and bonus points. The lesson is simple: Being sleep deprived puts you at risk for falling asleep unexpectedly.

Regardless of age, driving drowsy is like playing Russian roulette. As you fight off sleep, you may experience sudden, fleeting periods of microsleeps, where you fall asleep for a few brief seconds—long enough to create mayhem on the road. So if you are behind the wheel and feeling drowsy, pull over and let someone else drive. If you are alone, pull over and stop driving. If you find yourself reaching your destination but not remembering passing exits or other landmarks, you were asleep at the wheel—and are lucky to be alive.

Pregnancy's Effects on Sleep

A person's sleep can undergo significant changes during pregnancy. Early in a pregnancy, a person may find themselves sleeping more than usual, brought on, researchers believe, by rising levels of the hormone progesterone. Some may start feeling sleepier or more tired than usual even *before* they realize they are pregnant. Other physical changes, such as morning sickness, can also wear them out during this period. The second trimester is usually a better time for sleep, but sleep disruptions are typical in the third trimester. As a pregnant person's body changes, it may be difficult for them to sleep in their previously preferred position. Sleeping on their back or stomach will be challenging, and they may have to learn to sleep on their side. Pregnancy body pillows are designed to shift the pressure off the back and hips. Heartburn is also a common occurrence in pregnancy, especially if the person has had a tendency toward heartburn in the past. This can be helped by refraining from eating two hours before bed. That way, their stomach has had a chance to empty and they will be less likely to experience heartburn. They may also try sleeping in a more upright position. (For more on heartburn, see page 64.)

Two specific sleep disorders may flare up during pregnancy. The first is restless leg syndrome (RLS). As discussed on page 95, this syndrome is characterized by an uncomfortable urge to move, especially the legs. RLS is related to iron metabolism, and during pregnancy a person's iron stores can be depleted. It can be particularly bothersome in the second and third trimester. The sensation is worse in the evening and when sitting still and may improve with movement. (It also runs in families; if an otherwise healthy young child suffers from poor sleep due to "growing pains," I will ask if the parent had any unusual leg sensations during their pregnancy to help clinch the diagnosis.)

Obstructive sleep apnea may also develop during pregnancy. This further contributes to feelings of fatigue and can lead to dangerous increases in blood pressure. If a pregnant person starts to snore more, they should speak to their doctor about the possibility. Fortunately, modern treatments such as wearing a CPAP device can control obstructive sleep apnea and tamp down blood pressure spikes—see page 33.

Aside from the physical manifestations of pregnancy sleep, the uncertainties inherent in a pregnancy, particularly for a new parent, can result in restless nights. If a person has had prior bouts of insomnia before pregnancy, they may develop trepidation about how the pregnancy and ensuing parenting responsibilities will worsen their sleep. They may worry that if they do not get the rest they need they will not be a "good parent," putting further pressure upon themselves to sleep and causing them to fall into the classic insomniac worry trap (see page 45)—and potentially aggravating any postpartum depression. If you find during your pregnancy that your anxiety is affecting your sleep, or you're just not getting the restful sleep you need, consulting a sleep-medicine physician may be helpful.

Sleeping as You Age

The deep-sleep cycle known as slow-wave (N3) sleep is abundant in children; it may take several minutes to fully awaken a child in the middle of slow-wave sleep. By age sixty, slow-wave activity during sleep virtually disappears—particularly for men—so older adults wake up more often during the night. Some people may get up more often to urinate (in men's cases, because of prostate enlargement; in women's, bladder prolapse). Many elderly people get up at night to go to the bathroom because of medication side effects and undiagnosed obstructive sleep apnea, both treatable conditions. In addition, the tendency for sleep disorders may increase in older adults.

The amount you feel you need to sleep should stay mostly stable over time, but it often decreases with age. If you find you need *more* sleep with age, it could be a symptom of a serious health problem that requires evaluation. Consult your doctor, do not ignore it!

Menopause and Sleep

Poor sleep is a well-known feature of menopause. Especially in combination with estrogen, the hormone progesterone promotes sleep. These hormonal levels decrease in menopause, so it's no surprise that women are more likely to report difficulty falling and staying asleep during this transition. Menopause can also bring about obstructive sleep apnea. If after going through menopause, a woman finds herself snoring more, feeling more tired, or suffering from unexplained higher blood pressure, the possibility of obstructive sleep apnea should be considered. (See page 31 for more on this condition.)

Hormone replacement therapy (HRT) has been shown to improve sleep for menopausal women, but the decision to start this treatment must be made in consultation with a trusted health professional since it can have significant complications.

Even after other menopausal symptoms subside, sleep problems may persist and take on a life of their own. So many of the things that women find help them sleep better in the short run can make the problem worse down the road, such as drinking alcohol to help them nod off. Fortunately, this doesn't have to be the case. Many women of all ages sleep just fine. Seeing a sleep-medicine expert early on during menopause can help prevent years of poor sleep.

Now That I'm Retired, Can I Turn Off My Alarm Clock?

When people retire, they often think they can sleep in and wake up anytime they like. But the irregularity of their new sleep schedule often plants the seed for sleep problems.

One retiree came to me complaining of trouble falling asleep. When her husband passed away, she moved in with her younger sister, her sister's husband, and their adult children. Her sister and brother-in-law still worked and had to get up early in the morning, so she would go to her room after dinner so as not to bother them. She looked a little sad as she told me about this arrangement, and I wondered if she might be depressed. When I asked about her past employment, her face lit up. She told me she worked the overnight shift at a canning factory for twenty-five years. She loved her job and missed staying up late and singing while she worked. When I asked her to sing something, her sad expression changed to exuberance as she belted out a mariachi classic. It was beautiful to watch and listen to her. It turns out she was a natural night owl whose life circumstances had stopped her from doing what she loved. I suggested she find a choir or chorus that practiced at night. My patient left smiling.

If you slept well when you were employed, you may better enjoy your retirement if you resist the temptation to make big changes to your sleep patterns. Many patients who develop sleeping problems after retirement start to sleep better once they return to their prior schedule.

SEVEN

DREAMING: THE THEATER OF THE NIGHT

ARE OUR DREAMS random, or do they have some unconscious purpose? Despite thousands of years of speculation and now increasingly sophisticated research, the concept of an active unconscious mind is still being studied by scientists. But the answer is tantalizingly close and an important one: Unlocking this age-old question will likely lead us to understand the physiology of memory and creativity. In the pages that follow, we'll delve into this question as well as many others relating to the fascinating and mysterious act of dreaming.

Why Is It Hard to Remember Our Dreams?

If the fantastical events of our dreams occurred in real life, they would be hard to forget. Yet dreams are consistently difficult to recall. In order to remember a dream, you have to think about it while you're awake, often just as you're waking up (which is why some people put a pad and pencil next to their bed, so they can record their dreams before they forget them).

When you wake up people in the midst of REM sleep, however, there is about an 80 percent chance they will report a dream. This is because REM sleep is the time when you are most likely to be experiencing a dream (you can have fragments of sleep imagery during other stages of sleep, but not in the rich detail that REM dreams deliver). Even people who say they never dream will often report dreaming if they are awoken during this time.

In fact, dreams may be meant to be forgotten. REM sleep takes up about one to two hours of our nightly total sleep time. Imagine if every morning you had two hours' worth of vivid dreams to recount—you'd never get anything done! That dreams are hard to remember may be a clue to their potential function in the consolidation of memory (see opposite) as well as in understanding conditions such as dementia.

Why Are Dreams So Strange?

Dreams can be so vivid and detailed that you accept them as real experiences while they are happening. It's only when you awaken and remember fragments of your dreams that you realize how strange they actually are. When we are awake, the prefrontal cortex of our brain plays the role of the executive, filtering out irrelevant information in order to help us plan and make decisions. Other parts of our cerebral cortex also play a role in thinking while we are awake. As we enter REM sleep, the activity of the prefrontal cortex decreases, while in other parts of our neocortex activity increases. In the dream state, you are in an irrational world with its own peculiar logic. You are thinking differently. The miracle of dreaming is that the brain is creating a surreal world—and responding to it.

Dreams May Strengthen Our Memory

Our higher brain function allows us to adapt and thrive in a changing environment. It takes in and incorporates new information with what we already know to help us better understand the world around us. Any neural activity in the brain, like learning something new, must somehow change the memory networks in the brain: We need to connect our new memories with our old ones. At the same time, we need to forget things that aren't important. (If we remembered everything, our brain would likely be a lot less efficient!) This concept has been described by neuroscientist Matthew Walker. We probably do some of this reorganizing and learning while we're awake, but the restorative maintenance process of reorganizing our memories and resetting our brain functions happens on a larger scale while we sleep. This is why it can be so hard to think when we are tired and why our minds function so much better after a good night's sleep.

So far, it's hard to judge if the experience of having a dream is just a random by-product of some other neurological function or if it happens for a purpose, but some scientists believe that dreaming may be a part of the emotional and memory reprocessing that occurs during sleep. There is no doubt that when we dream we experience memories from our past. These memories must be activated or somehow brought forward into the brain activity that we experience as dreams. The basis of this approach, suggested by Dr. Robert Stickgold of Harvard, among others, is that dreaming is us experiencing the brain reactivating and modifying memories and emotions from earlier experiences. This would explain why we seem to commingle new and old memories in our dreams. If these theories are true, then dreaming is one of the mechanisms that our brain uses to improve our ability to adapt to our changing conscious world.

Dream research also suggests that memory functions are reflected in the actual content of dreams. In humans and rodents, patterns of neuronal firing that occur when learning a task while awake are reactivated during post-training sleep. In the hippocampus of rats, simultaneous recordings from large numbers of neurons have shown that specific patterns and neuronal firing sequences observed as the rats sought food on a circular track were replayed during subsequent sleep. In humans, positron emission tomography studies have shown that brain regions activated during the learning of a task were selectively reactivated during the next night's sleep. This supports the concept of sleep as an important part of memory consolidation. As Matthew Walker has said, "We dream to remember, and we dream to forget."

Dreams Enhance Our Creativity

Creativity is not only important to the arts; it also gives us tools to adapt to new environments and is a key component of problem-solving. Neuroscience is just now starting to understand the biological mechanisms by which the brain can have creative thoughts, and many of those mechanisms are at their best while we're asleep and dreaming.

When we are awake, we cannot ignore the world around us for very long. Our senses are constantly receiving new information that we must process and respond to quickly in the moment. When we are asleep, however, we disengage from the stimuli of the outside world. In the safety of our sleep, especially when we dream, our brains take the information we have been mulling over while we're awake and scan for connections to this material in other parts of our brain, which often results in new and potentially surreal combinations of thoughts. From this brew of neural activity during REM sleep, new ideas rise into our consciousness. If we manage to remember these thoughts, they can give us insights into the things we ruminate over when we are awake.

The Scary Art of Nightmares

If you were a painter and your artwork was frightening you, you might decide to change your painting style to create something less ominous. Think of nightmares as scary art your brain has created. Dreams come from the dreamer.

The first step in eliminating nightmares is to remove any external factors that may be disturbing your sleep. Anything that disrupts your sleep, including snoring, outside noises, and general discomfort, can wake you in the middle of a dream and thus make you more aware of its content. You can have nightmares if you go to sleep with too full a stomach and experience heartburn, for example—which is why some folks attribute nightmares to certain foods. If you are regularly having bad dreams, especially early in the night, don't eat anything for a couple of hours before going to bed.

Nightmares may also be a symptom of some physical ailment. Nightmares involving drowning or being buried alive, for example, may raise suspicions of obstructive sleep apnea, which makes it difficult to breathe while sleeping. Once the sleep apnea is corrected, the nightmares should quickly subside. (See page 31 for more on sleep apnea.)

If you can find nothing external disrupting your sleep and you still suffer from disturbing dreams or nightmares, you can actually learn to change your dreams. Two different techniques have been shown to work either alone or in combination: dream rehearsal and lucid dreaming. Dream rehearsal involves thinking about your recurring dreams while you're awake and imagining how they could play out differently. This can be done on your own or with the aid of a therapist. Lucid dreaming is a technique whereby you become aware that you are dreaming while remaining in the dream state. Turn to page 132 for more on these techniques.

Recurring Dreams Come from Recurring Thoughts

Most people have recurring dreams—the phenomenon of experiencing an element or a theme in your dreams over and over. Common themes include falling, flying, or being late. If dreams are important reflections of our thoughts and feelings, then it follows that having a recurring dream must have some meaning. Or not.

Dreams are hard to remember—unless, that is, you spend time while you're awake consciously reinforcing the memory of a dream. If you think about one of your dreams upon awakening, you are creating a conscious memory of that dream. That memory can then be reactivated in your sleep. So simply by creating a conscious memory of a dream, you're upping the chances of that dream recurring.

That said, recurring dreams *may* be an expression of unresolved emotional issues. The recurring imagery may even be information detritus stuck in some kind of loop. If the theory holds that dreaming is your brain processing and deleting information, excessively dwelling on recurring dreams is sort of like putting the trash out for collection, then deciding to carry the garbage back into your house.

If you're bothered by recurring dream content, try the dream rehearsal or lucid dreaming techniques outlined on the next page. A therapist can also help you explore any emotional issues that may be behind the constant rebooting of your dreams.

Rewrite Your Dreams

When you have a very scary dream, it is natural to want to avoid thinking about it. But when you are alone with your thoughts in bed, the memory of a nightmare may cause you to dread going to sleep. The less you sleep, the more pressure will build in your brain to go into REM sleep—the state in which it is most likely that your nightmares will recur. Break this cycle with a technique known as dream rehearsal. Think specifically about what is scaring you in your dreams and what would make it better. For example, if you are dreaming about being pinned down by a monster, visualize the monster becoming a snowman and melting away. Use your imagination and have fun coming up with alternative endings to your dreams—anything goes. Do this in the daytime, away from your bed. Then when it's time to go to sleep, remind yourself of the dream alternatives you came up with, and look forward to sleeping and dreaming. Keep reminding yourself that your dreams are your art, and you can change the artwork.

Control Your Dreams

In ordinary dreaming, the dreamer is forced to react to a world that feels out of their control. When we become aware that we are dreaming, however—while continuing to stay inside the dream—we can find ourselves in a world of our own creation whose only rules are the limits of our imagination. This is called lucid dreaming. The unique experience of actively controlling and manipulating our dreams is truly an altered state of consciousness. The art of lucid dreaming has been described in texts dating back to antiquity but became popularized in Western culture through the work of Dr. Stephen LaBerge.

Though many people report becoming aware they are dreaming while dreaming, lucid dreams are less common. Young people, in particular, report spontaneously having isolated lucid dreaming experiences, but studies show that true lucid dreamers represent just 10 percent of the population. The big question is: Can lucid dreaming be learned? There is no dearth of seminars, retreats, books, and online videos to learn and practice lucid dreaming. Even dietary supplements and various devices are sold to facilitate lucid dreaming—and more are in the pipeline. Any of these options may increase the chance of having a lucid dream, but not everyone can learn to predictably dream lucidly.

If you're interested in trying to learn to lucid dream, the first step is being able to recognize that the dream is a dream while you're in it. One technique to do this is called reality testing. Practice looking at something in detail several times a day—your hand, for example. Then when you are in a dream state, you may look at your hand and realize it is somehow different. This is a clue that lets you know you are in a dream. Perhaps the hardest part of lucid dreaming? Realizing your dream is a dream without waking yourself up. It can be startling! With practice, however, you may become used to the experience and be able to remain asleep. When that happens, you can start trying to manipulate the world inside your dream.

Do Animals Dream?

Probably yes, some do. We know that many mammals have the equivalent of REM sleep; it has also been shown to occur in experiments performed on birds, lizards, and even fish. In REM sleep, a signal from the brain stem puts us in a state of temporary paralysis, called REM atonia, which stops most of our muscles from moving. In experiments with cats, that signal was removed and the sleeping cats were observed moving and engaging in a range of complex behaviors independent of what was actually in front of them in the real world. Similar behavior was later seen in humans whose brain stem signal was malfunctioning. Those humans reported dream content that was consistent with their observed behaviors. It is safe to infer that the experimentally manipulated cats were acting based on some internal stimulation while in REM sleep—in other words, they were likely dreaming. If cats do it, then other animals can, too. We are not alone in our world of dreams.

EIGHT

SEEING A SLEEP DOCTOR

MILLIONS OF PEOPLE suffer needlessly from sleep disorders, yet the vast majority can find relief with the right approach. My experience shows that it is the rare person whose sleep does not improve when the problem is correctly addressed. If, after absorbing all the information in this book, you still have trouble sleeping, it may be time to see a sleep specialist.

Being a sleep-medicine physician is a fun gig compared with many other medical specialties, because most of my patients *actually get better*. Rarely a day goes by in the sleep clinic that I don't hear someone say how good they feel since they improved their sleep, and how they wished they had sought help sooner. In this final chapter, I'll take you on a virtual visit to the sleep clinic. I'll cover how to find the right doctor, questions to expect in your case history (and what your answers may mean), and what happens during a sleep study.

Finding the Right Doctor

If you tell your doctor you're tired most of the time, and your doctor says, "We're all tired," then it's time to get a new doctor.

Physicians are simply not taught enough about how to help people sleep better. Particularly given the time constraints of standard office visits, doctors are often reluctant to ask about patients' sleep habits, preferring to stay in their comfort zones and avoid "opening up a big can of worms." So sleep problems continue to be inadequately addressed, if they are addressed at all. This does not have to happen. If your sleep complaints persist and your doctor doesn't take the problem seriously, it's time to seek out a sleep-medicine physician.

It's critical that you see a *board-certified sleep specialist* in an *accredited sleep-medicine facility*. Many sleep-medicine clinics in operation in the United States are not accredited. When you make your appointment, confirm that the sleep clinic has been accredited by the American Academy of Sleep Medicine and that its doctors are board certified in sleep medicine. Many sleep-medicine physicians have medical training in other specialties; prior training in pulmonary medicine can be invaluable, because the most common reason a person seeks out a sleep consult is to test for obstructive sleep apnea. Some communities also have psychologists with specialized training in behavioral sleep medicine.

Visiting a Sleep Clinic

Clinical sleep medicine is modeled after other outpatient medical clinic encounters. As a new patient, you will be given paperwork to complete, including a questionnaire that focuses on your general health and explores your sleep history. You will then meet with a sleep physician who will take a detailed history of your concerns (see below). This is followed by a physical examination, which helps provide further information to support a preliminary diagnosis and develop a therapeutic plan. In the case of snoring or possible sleep apnea, the physical examination will focus on the throat, nose, and mouth—potential areas of obstruction. Physical evidence of heart disease, diabetes, or other chronic diseases will be considered.

It's a lot of information to share and consider, and a new patient visit shouldn't feel rushed. You may need to get confirmatory testing, such as blood work or X-rays. But most commonly, your diagnosis will involve a "sleep study" polysomnogram test to measure the quality of your sleep, described in detail on page 144.

Decoding Your Sleep History

A patient's sleep history is an invaluable diagnostic tool, especially when considering a diagnosis of chronic insomnia. I'll ask about the amount of sleep you average nightly, the perceived quality of your sleep, the timing of your sleep, and your state of mind when it comes to sleeping. I also want to know how you *feel*: How is your sleep different from the way you want, expect, or used to sleep? It's often helpful if a partner is on hand to confirm or flesh out a patient's story.

Following are five essential questions a doctor will ask while taking your sleep history, and what your answers may indicate.

1. **Do you have trouble falling asleep, staying asleep, or both?**

   Having difficulty falling asleep is an easier problem to fix than difficulty staying asleep, especially if a patient is motivated to make some lifestyle changes. When someone is having difficulty falling asleep, a doctor will typically recommend a later bedtime paired with a fixed wake-up time, along with changes to lifestyle factors such as late-in-the-day caffeine use.

   Older patients and those with many years of poor sleep are more likely to have trouble staying asleep. This is typical in chronic insomnia. These patients often suffer from hypervigilance around sleep, and they greatly benefit from the strategies outlined in Sleep for the Insomniac, beginning on page 39.

   When patients do not have trouble falling asleep but wake up several times during the night and are able to get back to sleep relatively quickly (say, in less than five minutes), the situation is more likely due to a physical interruption of their sleep, such as chronic pain or periodic limb movement disorder.

2. **How did the problem start, how long has this been an issue, and what do you think may be driving it?**

People don't immediately rush to see a sleep doctor after a few nights of poor sleep. They often turn first to friends and family for advice—and sometimes for more than advice (like sleep medications). Usually whatever seems to have triggered the poor sleep will pass, and they will start sleeping better again. Down the road, if something triggers another bout of insomnia, they'll try whatever worked before. It might succeed again, cementing the idea that they've found the solution. But if another bout of insomnia happens and the strategies they've tried before no longer do the trick, they'll try something new. Even though insomnia patterns can wax and wane over time, eventually the bouts of insomnia may build, with the periods of good sleep growing shorter, until insomnia dominates their nighttime. Every now and then they might get a good night of sleep—a relief, but also vexing in the patient's quest for why they sleep well on some nights and not on others. Determining where someone is in this process can help get to the heart of what is driving their insomnia. Then we can explore why previous treatments failed and pinpoint treatments that *will* work.

3. **Do you look forward to sleeping? Or do you see it as a hassle or an inconvenience?**

For some people, going to sleep is the best part of their day; for others the worst; and for most of us, it's just part of the daily routine. I need to know how patients think about sleep and *why* they want to sleep. For example, do you see sleep as a restorative process or an escape from an unhappy life? Do you see it as a well-earned break from your responsibilities? Or do you consider sleep a necessary inconvenience?

If a person suffers from poor sleep but looks forward to sleeping, I'm more likely to consider physical causes. If a person describes dread at the thought of going to sleep, I consider possible psychological issues such as trauma or negative conditioning or associations around sleep.

4. In the past, what did you consider good sleep?

The answer to this question gives us a target to aim for. If you enjoyed an average of seven hours of sleep most of your adult life but are now sleeping only six and want to get eight, I would suggest that you set the more realistic goal of returning to seven hours of sleep per night. If you blame your snoring on a weight gain, I ask if you snored when you weighed less. If the answer is no, then getting back to your original weight may be a useful goal. When retired patients complain about poor sleep, I ask about their sleep schedules when they worked and felt they slept better (for more on this, see page 124).

5. Do you sleep differently in different locations?

One of the interesting things we routinely see in sleep studies is that people wearing wires and sensors attached to their bodies, sleeping in a bedroom they've never slept in—with cameras pointing at them and strangers walking into their room the next morning—can report a great night's sleep. But they do, over and over. People with insomnia can be so conditioned to sleeping poorly in their own home that they sleep better pretty much anywhere other than in their own bed.

A patient of mine was having trouble sleeping since he had inherited his family's fortune. He felt great responsibility in managing the money his family had entrusted him with, and his bed was scattered with financial statements that he would review as he fell asleep at night. He was using the bed to *work*, not sleep. Once he moved his paperwork out of the bedroom, he started sleeping better. I see similar patterns with graduate students working on their thesis. School papers litter their bedrooms, a constant reminder of unfinished work. It's no wonder they have trouble sleeping in that stressful environment!

Your bedroom should be a place of serenity and security. Study or work elsewhere, and take back your ultimate sanctuary for the health of your sleep.

Those five questions are the basics. I also widen the scope of the sleep history, asking questions like the following about outside factors and behavioral habits that may be impeding sleep:

- **Household situation.** In order to help a person sleep better, I need to understand the sleep dynamics in the home. I want to know how other family members or roommates sleep; if you share your sleep environment with a partner, children, or pets; if you are taking care of other adults in the home; and any other social factors that are keeping you from sleeping well. A number of people feel guilty admitting they sleep better when their partners are away. If that is the case, the bed partner may have sleep problems that have not been addressed that are disturbing the patient's sleep. Perhaps the couple has very different sleep habits or schedules that are in conflict. There could even be interpersonal issues that are interrupting the patient's sleep that need to be explored. Pets in the bedroom can also be a contentious issue, especially if allergies emerge (or the pet "belongs" to just one person in the relationship).

- **Sleep location.** I never assume a person always sleeps in a bed in a bedroom. Some people fall asleep in one part of the home and then wake up and move to another room. You may be the first one to fall asleep, but then your bed partner's snoring chases you out of bed. I've lost count of the number of big men who tell me they spend many nights in a too-small child's bed when their kids climb into the parents' bed in the middle of the night.

- **Sleep schedule.** What is your typical sleep schedule? How is it different on workdays and days off or vacations? Sleeping in more than two hours on weekends is a sign of potentially significant sleep deprivation during the workweek. Being a shift worker or having flexible work hours can cause sleep issues, too. When second- or third-shift workers try to sleep in a pattern that aligns closer to the rest of their family on their days off, the ensuing sleep-schedule shifts can wreak havoc with their circadian rhythms. People who seem best able to navigate these schedules usually keep a similar schedule on their days off, or they have worked out a routine where they break up their sleep into two segments to accommodate their family and work demands. (And as we get older it gets harder to adapt to shifting our schedules, which is why people complain of "burning out" on shift-work positions.)

- **Stressors.** Do you feel safe in your home? Sometimes people describe such stressful life situations that I point out it would be odd if they slept well.

- **Medication, caffeine, and alcohol.** What, if any, medications—including prescription, over the counter, and supplements—have you tried? What was your experience with them? I will also ask about caffeine and alcohol use.

- **Health issues.** Finally, I ask about allergies and any pertinent family medical history. Sleep disorders like restless leg syndrome tend to run in the family. I also delve into people's mental health history, such as if they've ever been treated for depression or suicidal thoughts. I'll consider external health factors, too, such as pet dander, that may be found in the home.

The Sleep Study

There are myriad ways to measure the quality of a person's sleep, and new technology is emerging to add to physicians' diagnostic options. The classic, and most common, way to measure sleep quality is with an all-night sleep recording, called a polysomnogram.

A polysomnogram is carried out in a sleep center or sleep laboratory. You will typically be asked to arrive at the center after dinner, where you'll change into sleep clothes. The clinic will provide a comfortable sleep environment, with soundproofing, clean bedding, individual temperature controls, and shower facilities (you will likely want to shower after the study, to wash off any glue from the sensors). You should be able to go straight to work the next morning, if you wish.

Once you are comfortably in bed, technologists will attach several sensors to your body that measure brain waves, eye movements, body movements, muscle tone, breathing patterns, oxygen levels, and heart rhythm. The entire time you are sleeping in the lab, a trained technologist will be observing you via remote infrared cameras and will be able to intervene if any of the sensors fall off or if you need assistance.

Dozens of measurements are obtained from the all-night sleep recording. The recording is processed by another sleep technologist, who will score the various sleep stages and tabulate any abnormal breathing, cardiac, brain-wave, or motor events. The study will determine how much you actually slept relative to the time you were in bed, how long it took you to fall asleep (sleep latency), how long it took for you to reach your first REM/dreaming episode (REM latency), and how much deep sleep and light sleep were present. (Interestingly, some sleep-study participants who claim they did not sleep at all clearly did so during the study.)

A sleep study can identify what is causing a person to wake up during the night, such as trouble breathing or abnormal body movements. It can also determine if violent behavior in sleep is coming out of REM sleep or slow-wave (N3) sleep, a distinction that is important for both diagnosis and treatment. That said, a sleep study is only a snapshot of one night. False negative results can occur—for example, if a person barely sleeps—which can necessitate repeating the study.

Technology now makes it possible to perform a sleep study in your own home. Some home sleep tests can be mailed straight to your door; you simply mail the test back when it's completed. The advantages of a home sleep study over a traditional sleep-lab study are that it is less expensive and more convenient; there are a number of disadvantages, however. You are not attended by trained sleep technologists, so if a sensor falls off or something malfunctions, no one is there to troubleshoot the problem in real time. Home sleep studies record fewer channels of information and generally have a narrow focus, designed mainly to recognize sleep apnea events, so if a patient has a problem with seizures, elevated carbon dioxide levels, or abnormal body movements such as leg kicks or sleepwalking, the home sleep test will not pick it up. Home sleep studies also tend to underreport the severity of sleep apnea: A false negative result may necessitate either repeating the home sleep test or doing a more comprehensive in-lab sleep study. An attended in-lab sleep study is also better for people with a severe degree of sleep apnea, because the technologist can spend the first portion of the night confirming the diagnosis and the latter part trying out different treatment options. Finally, home sleep studies have not been well validated for use in children being evaluated for sleep disorders. All of that said, sometimes an at-home sleep study is the best option available to you, such as if you live prohibitively far from an accredited sleep clinic, are home-bound for any reason, or if an in-lab sleep study is otherwise unavailable.

In the end, sleep studies, whether done in the home or in an accredited sleep center, are just diagnostic tools. What is most important is the skill of the clinician in interpreting your results.

The Follow-Up

The most critical part of a sleep evaluation is the follow-up. After the evaluation is completed and the therapeutic plan is established, it is essential for you and your sleep clinician to meet again, to see if your issues have been adequately addressed and whether things have changed.

Further complicating a sleep evaluation is that you may suffer from more than one sleep disorder, and one disorder can set off another. For example, those with obstructive sleep apnea often suffer from breathing problems that wake them up at night. These frequent awakenings can lead to maladaptive sleep habits that then lead to chronic insomnia. The good news is that board-certified sleep-medicine specialists are equipped to parse out your various sleep problems and help you sleep better for a healthier life.

FINAL THOUGHTS

Modern sleep science has come a long way in a very short time. The true promise of sleep is that we all live healthier, longer, and more enjoyable lives when we sleep well. It is the ultimate form of self-care, and it begins with making quality sleep a priority. Societal pressures to rob us of sleep may feel relentless, but as sleep science advances and we all learn to value our sleep health, the future looks promising indeed. The new reality is that we no longer need to wake up feeling tired—our very health depends on it. I hope this book has helped you understand that you and your loved ones can all sleep better.

RESOURCES

RESOURCES

CDC.gov/sleep
The Centers for Disease Control and Prevention offers information and resources regarding sleep and sleep disorders, as well as on the importance of sleep for the nation's overall health.

sleepeducation.org
This public-education website from the American Academy of Sleep Medicine helps you locate an accredited sleep-medicine clinic within your zip code.

startschoollater.net
This website, from the nonprofit organization Start School Later, provides materials and information for any individual or group that wants to advocate for later start times for schools, to allow students to get more sleep and to lead healthier lives.

thensf.org
The National Sleep Foundation is a nonprofit public health organization that advocates for healthy sleep. Its website is a good resource for general information about sleep and its impact on society.

FURTHER READING

FURTHER READING

Dement's Sleep and Dreams by Rafael Pelayo and William C. Dement
The first college-level sleep textbook, and the core text for Stanford University's Sleep and Dreams course.

Lucid Dreaming by Stephen LaBerge
This is the original how-to manual on training yourself to lucid dream.

The Promise of Sleep by William C. Dement
The pioneer of sleep medicine lays out his vision for a healthier life.

Quiet Your Mind and Get to Sleep by Colleen Carney, Ph.D., and Rachel Manber, Ph.D.
This workbook guides readers through behavioral treatment of insomnia.

Why We Sleep by Matthew Walker
A brilliant Berkeley neuroscientist explains the basic mechanisms of sleep and its implications for our health.

GLOSSARY

apnea-hypopnea index (AHI) The total number of apneas (cessation of breathing) and hypopneas (episodes of shallow breathing that disrupt sleep) during the night divided by the total hours of sleep.

biological clock *See* circadian clock.

Brown noise Consistent, machine-generated sounds designed to mask disruptive sonic shifts; high-frequency sound waves are filtered out, making the tones lower and deeper than white noise.

chronic insomnia Episodes of sleeplessness that occur repeatedly and that can persist for at least three months and often for years.

circadian clock A tiny cluster of neurons in the brain that synchronizes the body's sleep and walk rhythms. Also known as the biological clock.

circadian system The biological process that allows our bodies to synchronize our internal rhythms with the external twenty-four-hour light cycle.

cognitive behavioral therapy for insomnia (CBT-I) A form of therapy that treats insomnia by helping people change the thoughts and behaviors that cause or worsen sleep problems.

complete sleep deprivation Going longer than twenty-four hours without sleep.

CPAP (continuous positive airway pressure) machine A bedside device used to treat obstructive sleep apnea that forces positive air pressure through the user's nose, causing the user's throat to remain open.

delayed sleep phase syndrome (DSPS) A circadian sleep disorder characterized by difficulty falling asleep without difficulty staying asleep.

dream rehearsal A therapeutic approach to thinking about recurring dreams while awake and imagining how they could play out differently.

Ferber method A behavioral technique to help infants sleep without disrupting the parents' sleep by teaching them to self-soothe within a structured schedule that can include allowing infants to cry for a predetermined amount of time without the parents' intervention. This is sometimes referred to as a type of "sleep training."

hypnic jerks (sleep starts) Sudden, uncontrolled, and brief contractions of the body or the limbs that can occur when one is transitioning from being awake into sleep.

hypnotics Medications to help a person sleep, often referred to as prescription sleeping pills.

insomnia Trouble falling asleep and/or staying asleep, resulting in some form of daytime impairment. *See* chronic insomnia, transient insomnia.

K-complexes A large waveform that may be seen on an electroencephalogram (EEG) during stage 2 of NREM sleep. K-complexes seem to help a person stay asleep and also aid in memory consolidation.

lucid dreaming To become aware that you are dreaming while remaining in the dream state.

microsleeps Very brief bouts of unintended sleep in which a person may not realize they are asleep.

narcolepsy A neurological disorder that usually begins in adolescence or young adulthood and is marked by excessive daytime sleepiness and REM–like phenomena while awake, including sleep paralysis, cataplexy, and hallucinations.

nocturnal lagophthalmos The inability to close the eyelids while sleeping.

non–rapid eye movement (NREM) sleep The bulk of human sleep and the period that is not associated with vivid dreaming. It is divided into three stages: N1 (light sleep), in which we transition from the awake state into sleep; N2 (intermediate sleep), which takes up about half of our total sleep time; and N3 (commonly referred to as slow-wave sleep), which is our deepest sleep, taking up 10 percent or less of total adult sleep time.

obstructive sleep apnea The interruption of breathing during sleep due to a temporary blockage of the throat; a potentially dangerous sleep disorder.

periodic limb movement disorder (PLMD) A sleep disorder in which one moves their limbs, typically the legs, in a repetitive pattern while asleep.

pink noise Consistent, machine-generated sounds designed to mask disruptive sonic shifts; mid-frequency sound waves are filtered out, making it deeper than white noise but less deep than Brown noise.

polysomnogram (PSG) An all-night sleep recording that measures a person's brain waves, eye movements, body movements, muscle tone, breathing patterns, oxygen levels, and heart rhythm, as well as any other additional signals of interest.

rapid eye movement (REM) sleep The period of sleep in which the sleeping brain is most active, the majority of dreaming occurs, and the eyes jerk in different directions, among other physical effects. It occupies about 20 percent of sleep time. It was named by Dr. William C. Dement.

REM latency How long it takes to reach the first REM/dreaming episode, usually measured in minutes.

REM pressure The increase in the amount and intensity of REM sleep in response to REM deprivation.

second sleep The habit of breaking nighttime sleep into two parts, with a period of activity in between. Part of the spectrum of polyphasic sleep patterns.

sleep apnea Cessation of breathing for ten seconds or more during sleep. *See* obstructive sleep apnea.

sleep architecture The repetitive pattern of the combination of sleep stages and cycles.

sleep bruxism The grinding of one's teeth during sleep.

sleep cycle A period of time, lasting about ninety minutes, that includes the various sleep stages and repeats throughout the night. *See* sleep stages.

sleep debt The accumulated deficit of sleep that occurs when someone doesn't meet their daily sleep requirement.

sleep drunkenness The sluggish sensation felt upon awakening after a prolonged period of sleep. *See* sleep inertia.

sleep fragmentation When sleep cycles are disrupted.

sleep hygiene Recommendations for things to avoid in the hopes of improving sleep quality, popularized by Dr. Peter Hauri.

sleep inertia Feeling groggy, achy, or listless upon awakening.

sleep latency The length of time it takes to fall asleep.

sleep paralysis A temporary inability to move while falling asleep or upon waking.

sleep restriction A behavioral technique within cognitive behavioral therapy for insomnia that improves the ability to stay asleep by dictating a narrow window of time that someone actually spends in bed.

sleep spindles An electroencephalography (EEG) pattern consisting of sinusoidal bursts of activity, lasting from a half to several seconds, originating from the thalamus. Sleep spindles may play a role in the formation of memories.

sleep stages There are two basic types of sleep in humans: REM and NREM. NREM is further divided into three stages (N1, N2, and N3) based on predictable cycles of various electrical brainwave patterns.

sleep study Any extended clinical measurement of a person's sleep. This is usually performed overnight in a medical facility, but can also be done in a person's home. Sleep studies are typically used to measure sleep quality and detect disruptions of a person's sleep. *See* polysomnogram (PSG).

sleep terrors An abnormal event characterized by a sleeping person suddenly sitting up and letting out a bloodcurdling scream. This is most common in young children and tends to occur in the first third of the night.

sleeping aid Substances used and marketed to help remedy sleep problems such as transient insomnia. These are often available without a prescription.

sleepwalking A sleep disorder classified under the category of parasomnias whereby a person may carry out a wide range of behaviors while remaining in a deep sleep.

slow-wave sleep Another name for the N3 period of NREM sleep.

somniloquy Talking in one's sleep.

stimulus control A behavioral technique within cognitive behavioral therapy for insomnia that promotes more predictable sleep by helping one to form positive associations with the sleep environment (such as the bedroom).

transient insomnia A short-term inability to sleep well that generally lasts only a few nights and for which the cause is usually apparent.

white noise A machine-generated sound made up of all audible frequencies at the same intensity. *See also* Brown noise, pink noise.

ACKNOWLEDGMENTS

There are many people to thank for creating *How to Sleep*. This book originated with Katherine "Kitty" Cowles, who reached out to Erin Digitale at Stanford to identify a potential author for a book on sleep. Fortunately, Erin and Lisa Kim recommended me. From that connection, Kitty led me to meet my editor, Bridget Monroe Itkin, at Artisan Books. I didn't really appreciate what a book editor did until I met Bridget. Now I know what a good editor can do—she helped me visualize what this book would become. The team at Artisan that helped create *How to Sleep* includes its publisher and editorial director Lia Ronnen, along with Carson Lombardi, Elise Ramsbottom, Nina Simoneaux, Suet Chong, Nancy Murray, Erica Huang, Allison McGeehon, Theresa Collier, Amy Michelson, and Patrick Thedinga. Thank you all, and I hope you are sleeping well.

Alexis Lipsitz received a manuscript full of run-on sentences, redundancies, poor grammar, and general gibberish and turned it into prose. I know that was not easy. Thank you!

I am grateful to my mentors who taught me how to be a sleep-medicine physician, starting with Dr. Michael Thorpy at Montefiore Medical Center. Without Michael, I would never have gotten to Stanford and become privileged to learn directly from the original sleep-medicine physicians, Drs. Christian Guilleminault and William "Bill" Dement. Bill graciously and generously has allowed me to continue his tradition of teaching Stanford students the importance of sleep. Dr. Sharon Keenan patiently provided me the space to learn how to share this information.

My wife and children have encouraged and supported me throughout this process. They are the ones who motivate me to get out of bed in the morning. I love you.

Ultimately, there would be no book if my patients had not taught me so much. Thousands have trusted me to be their physician. I can never thank them enough.

INDEX